A
WOMAN'S
WAY
through
THE
TWELVE
STEPS

Other Publications by Stephanie S. Covington, Ph.D.

Awakening Your Sexuality: A Guide for Recovering Women

Beyond Trauma: A Healing Journey for Women
(facilitator's guide, workbook, and DVDs)

Helping Women Recover: A Program for Treating Addiction
(facilitator's guide and woman's journal)

Helping Women Recover: A Program for Treating Substance Abuse
(special edition for use in the criminal justice system)

Leaving the Enchanted Forest:
The Path from Relationship Addiction to Intimacy

Voices: A Program of Self-Discovery and Empowerment for Girls
(facilitator guide and journal)

A Woman's Way through the Twelve Steps: Program DVD

A Woman's Way through the Twelve Steps Facilitator's Guide

A Woman's Way through the Twelve Steps Workbook

Women and Addiction: A Gender-Responsive Approach
(manual, DVD, and CE test)

Women in Recovery: Understanding Addiction
(also available in Spanish)

A WOMAN'S WAY

through

THE TWELVE STEPS

Stephanie S. Covington, Ph.D.

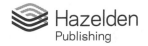

Hazelden
Publishing

Hazelden Publishing
Center City, Minnesota 55012
hazelden.org/bookstore

Library of Congress Cataloging-in-Publication Data
Covington, Stephanie.
    A Woman's way through the twelve steps/Stephanie S. Covington.
        p.   cm.
    Includes bibliographical references.
    ISBN 13: 978-0-89486-993-8
    ISBN 10: 0-89486-993-0
    1. Obsessive-compulsive disorder—Treatment. 2. Twelve-step programs. 3. Women—Mental health. I. Title.
RC533.C68 1994
362.29' 186'082—dc20   94-22135
                                                                  CIP

Editor's note
The Twelve Steps are reprinted and adapted with permission of Alcoholics Anonymous World Services, Inc. Permission to reprint and adapt the Twelve Steps does not mean that AA has reviewed or approved the contents of this publication, nor that AA agrees with the views expressed herein. AA is a program of recovery from alcoholism *only*–use of the Twelve Steps in connection with programs and activities that are patterned after AA, but that address other problems, does not imply otherwise.

Contents

Acknowledgments

WRITING THIS BOOK was a privilege. The pages are filled with the words and experiences of many recovering women, and I found it deeply rewarding and meaningful to listen to their stories.

There are many people who have helped to create this book and make it a reality. I am grateful to the many friends and colleagues who have quietly supported me—and more importantly, supported this book by encouraging me and offering their belief in the value, worth, and necessity of this book.

A special thanks to my editorial consultant and good friend, Roy M. Carlisle of Mills House, whose support, encouragement, and expertise are indispensable.

Sid Farrar, Judy Delaney, and Darlene Gish at Hazelden have been enthusiastic and supportive throughout the life of this project. Don Freeman and Caryn Pernu have thoughtfully managed the production details with expertise and ease.

The various versions and revisions of each chapter were created with the help of Lisa Raleigh, Debra Sands Miller, Shirley Loffer, and Judy Delaney. Thank you for sharing your talents.

I am also grateful to Penny Philpot. Her wisdom, insight, humor, and companionship have nourished me tremendously.

I feel a deep sense of gratitude for all of you.

Special Acknowledgments

A SPECIAL THANK-YOU TO THE WOMEN who were interviewed for this book: Donna B., Rhonda C., Sylvia C., Lori D., Tryshe D., Kathryn D. F., Anne G., Jane G., Susan G., Beverly H., Carter H., Donna H., Judi H., Nicole J., Charlotte K., Jean K., Jessica M., Irene P., Chandra S., and Janet S.

In the tradition of the Twelve Step programs, they remain anonymous. However, their life stories are rich in their diversity— reflecting differences in age, race, class, ethnicity, religion, geographic location, occupation, choice of partner, and role as mother.

Throughout the pages of this book, these women share their experience, strength, and hope. Their voices reflect their "principles, not personalities."

Together they represent over 320 years of sobriety/abstinence in AA, OA, NA, Alanon, and Debtors Anonymous.

Thank you for sharing your wisdom and your vision for women's health and healing.

The stories in this book are true, but names and identifying details have been changed to protect the anonymity of the women interviewed.

Introduction

As a woman in a Twelve Step recovery program, or as one who is beginning to think about recovery from addiction, you may be thrilled to find a book that focuses on your issues as a woman in recovery. Or you may be wondering what this book offers that you have not found in other books or in Twelve Step literature and meetings.

Through my own recovery from alcoholism and my professional and personal relationships with women in recovery from a variety of addictions, I have found that a number of issues unique to women are overlooked in most Twelve Step programs. Some of these issues include the effects on women of the language of the Twelve Steps, the psychological development of women as it relates to addiction and recovery, and the social and cultural factors that affect us as women—both in general as females in a male-dominated society and specifically as women living through addiction and recovery.

As a result of these omissions, many of us have struggled to stay with a recovery program that does not completely meet our needs or match our values. Others may have experienced relapse and felt that something was missing from their recovery program without being able to identify what that something was.

My hope is that this book will offer you a new, more accessible perspective on recovery from addiction, one that acknowledges your needs and concerns as a woman. This new perspective is based on a more open exploration and a more flexible interpretation of the Twelve Steps as they relate to women in recovery. It derives from the mutual learning that is possible among women as we share the stories of our struggles and triumphs in recovery. My hope is that this perspective will empower you to take ownership of your recovery process as well as your growth as a woman.

The Twelve Steps were first developed in 1939 by the founders of Alcoholics Anonymous (AA). In the past fifty-five years, the Steps have been adopted by a variety of self-help groups and have provided an invaluable resource and guide for people on the recovery journey. Millions have taken this journey, using the spiritual, emotional, and practical resources of the Twelve Steps in their recovery from alcoholism, drug dependency, eating disorders, sexual compulsions, gambling, and more.

The history and tradition of the Twelve Steps provide a sense of security and certainty about their effectiveness. At the same time, it is important to recognize that the Steps were written by men for men's needs in recovery at a time when women had few resources and little social, political, or economic power. At the time the Steps were written, the possibility of a woman becoming addicted was barely considered and women with addictions faced shunning and secrecy.

As more and more women have entered recovery programs over the last twenty years, we have found that recovery may mean something different for us as women. Even more, we are finding that the journey of recovery is unique for each of us as individuals: there is no right or wrong way to proceed in "working" the Steps. As you read this book and explore the meaning and practice of the Twelve

Steps, you will find many different perspectives on each Step to help you create your own path in your journey to recovery.

Using the Steps as guides, you will rediscover what you think, feel, and believe, and then begin to connect this with your actions with other people in the world around you. This experience of connecting your feelings and beliefs with your actions is what I call wholeness, or integrity.

You will come back to this theme of unifying your inner and outer life throughout the journey. Each of the Twelve Steps in some way touches upon it because all of the Steps involve soul-searching and self-honesty. Ultimately, the underlying theme of the Steps is living a life that is consistent with your deepest values. The Steps are designed to help you discover what those values are—to look at your inner life—so that you can see how you may be acting contrary to your values and learn to honor them in the future—in your outer life. This is what recovery is about: integrating inner with outer and thereby creating integrity.

As you turn inward you will need to search deeply so that you can use the Steps in a meaningful way. Because the Steps were written in 1939 by men for male alcoholics, the language of the Steps may appear to have little relevance for you as a contemporary woman. While much of the AA literature has been revised and updated, the Twelve Steps themselves still appear in their original wording. Consequently, when you read the Steps today, they may rightfully seem to be from another era.

Of course, many women have no problem with the Steps as written, but a significant number of women take issue with the language of the Steps, viewing it as exclusive and sexist. This book is intended, then, to make the Steps more inclusive, more accessible to women, to speak more directly to the ways women experience addiction and recovery, as well as everyday life. It can be used as a companion to the *Twelve Steps and Twelve Traditions* or by itself.

There have been many efforts to rewrite the Steps from a woman's point of view, but often a rewritten version of the Steps moves too far away from the original spirit of the program. Having spoken of the limitations of Twelve Step programs, it is equally important to acknowledge the many ways in which the spirit of these programs meets the needs and concerns of women.

Perhaps most important for women is that recovery takes place not in isolation, but in connection with others in recovery. AA is the model for mutual-help programs. It is in this mutuality—the open sharing of feelings, struggles, hopes, and triumphs without blame or judgment—that women can find the most powerful resources for healing.

The lack of a hierarchical structure in Twelve Step programs is also attractive to women, many of whom have experienced the abuses of traditional top-down power structures. In Twelve Step programs, there are no experts or supervisors or financial backers to exercise authority over program members. Each member is viewed as a potential contributor to the support and recovery of all other members.

Also important to women, many of whom may lack financial and other resources, is the accessibility of Twelve Step meetings. They are free, open to all who are in need, and, especially in urban areas, readily available in terms of both location and time of day.

In many ways, Twelve Step recovery programs are based on a feminine model of support and healing. Although the language and practices may not always follow this feminine model, the spirit of the Steps and the structure of Twelve Step programs offer an opportunity for us to explore both our recovery from addiction and our empowerment as women.

Rather than rewrite the Steps in a way that attempts to fit all women, we can instead work with the original Steps—paying close attention to the spirit and meaning—and reinterpret the language to support our own recovery. As Ruth, a recovering alcoholic and bulimic says, "The program defies the language." In other words, there's something powerful and healing concealed beneath the archaic wording of the Steps. When we look inside ourselves and reframe the original wording in the way that works best for us, each of us, individually, can discover the meaning for ourselves.

Still, recovery is not a solitary process. There's no expectation that we will read program materials in solitude, reflect on them, and independently arrive at our own personalized interpretations. Instead, we are supported by others in the Twelve Step tradition: sharing experience, strength, and hope. In Twelve Step programs, there is an ongoing and deep interchange of personal information. Other people will share their stories and they will hear ours. We learn from each other.

In that spirit, this book offers the stories of many women who have traveled through and around the Steps, have thoughtfully examined the language and the concepts, and—listening to both their inner wisdom and the outer voices of the women around them in recovery—have discovered what fits for them and what doesn't. Theirs are not the voices of authority, but simply the voices of other recovering women, like you, who have created for themselves a personal, feminine interpretation of the Twelve Steps.

Author's Note about the Cover Design

THIS BOOK'S NEW COVER DESIGN (done in 2009) features the lotus flower. A picture of a lotus can be a meaningful and powerful symbol for women's recovery. The lotus rises from muddy waters to blossom. Although it grows with its roots deep in the mud, it emerges pure and unblemished. It unfolds gradually, one petal at a time, to blossom in the sunlight.

The mud can symbolize murky beginnings, the material world, or the darkness of addiction. The water can symbolize experience, transition, or recovery. The lotus can symbolize the purity of the soul, rebirth, spiritual awakening, and enlightenment. For thousands of years, the lotus has been associated with spiritual practices in many religious traditions. It also symbolizes detachment from worldly desires and illusions.

I see the lotus as a symbol of women's recovery. Recovery is a transformational experience. When a woman recovers, she is able to say, "Who I am today is not who I was." The elegant and beautiful lotus flower that emerges from the mud is the beautiful woman within.

The Step Before the Steps

THE JOURNEY THROUGH THE TWELVE STEPS often involves a pre-step—a "step before the Steps," if you will. In this step before, "we concede to ourselves that we are alcoholic"[1] (or suffering from another addiction). If you are not yet ready to concede that addiction is the problem, you might be ready to admit that some areas of your life are chaotic or out of control.

For many of us there is a growing awareness that things must change. As this feeling gets stronger, we find we are ready to take this pre-step: to admit that we need help and to accept help when it is offered, even if we didn't seek it. Then we find ourselves on the recovery journey.

The first part of the journey takes us through the Twelve Steps from a woman's perspective. We will explore how the Steps help us overcome addictions and work to heal and change ourselves, creating the possibility of a new and different life. Part of the surprising truth about recovery is that our ability to use the Twelve Steps and to apply them to other areas of our lives grows as our journey progresses. So, as we go on, we will explore the four areas of life where recovering women say they experience the most change—self, relationship, sexuality, and spirituality.

Step One

We admitted we were powerless over alcohol—
that our lives had become unmanageable.

We ALL KNOW THE SAYING that each journey begins with the first step. Each of us has taken many first steps in our lives—leaving home, going to school, starting a job, getting married, beginning a family. And each of us knows the many feelings that arise with these first steps—doubt, confusion, fear, relief, joy, sadness, and more.

Taking the first step in recovery may bring many of these same feelings. These are natural and even expected feelings any time we start something new. Many women like us have taken this first step in recovery no matter how difficult or frightening it seemed, and each of us has received many benefits, over time, from our efforts.

Recovery begins with Step One, when we admit that we're powerless over alcohol, and that as a result, our lives are unmanageable.*

---

*While Step One reads "powerless over alchohol," we can be powerless over any behavior we can't stop or control. The Twelve Steps of AA have been adapted and used successfully by people struggling with many kinds of addictive behaviors. You can substitute words such as *drugs, food, sex, money, gambling,* or *relationships* for the word *alcohol.*

After reading this first Step, you may wonder how it could possibly apply to you. Do you have a sense of how little power you have over the way you drink or use drugs? Are you able to see unmanageability in your life? Have you tried to control your addiction without success?

For some women this Step makes perfect sense. It is a simple act of admitting what we already know to be true—we can't control our drinking or using. It is obvious to us that our lives are out of control and unmanageable.

I remember feeling a vague sense of comfort when I read Step One. Admitting my powerlessness over alcohol gave me a sense of relief and reassurance. I finally understood why my attempts to control my drinking had not worked. Not being able to control my drinking meant I was addicted to alcohol! Only when I acknowledged that I had no power at all over my drinking was I able to start making sense of the difficulties in my life. This understanding of Step One gave me a sense of hope.

For others beginning recovery, it can be much harder to recognize powerlessness and unmanageability. This acknowledgment can be particularly challenging for those of us who have continued to maintain our commitments and responsibilities in spite of our addiction.

Some of us feel that Step One asks more of us than we expected. We enter recovery wanting only to change the way we drink or use drugs. Or we want *more* control over our lives, not less. And no matter what our situation, thinking of ourselves as powerless or out of control can feel very threatening and uncomfortable.

It is common to wonder how a Twelve Step program, and Step One in particular, is going to make a difference in our lives. Yet

Step One tells us there is a surprising solution: only when we realize we *can't* control our drinking or drug use or eating, do we find a way to change. Letting go of the illusion that we can control our addictive behavior is the first Step on the journey of recovery.

THE ENDLESS LOOP OF ADDICTION

One way to let go of our illusion of control and begin to recognize our powerlessness is to look at the endless cycle of our addiction. We use alcohol or drugs (or food or relationships) to change how we feel—to numb our pain or to feel better about ourselves or to forget our problems. But the change is only temporary. Reality swiftly returns when we wake up the next morning with the same feelings and the same problems—along with a hangover and perhaps guilt about what we had done while drinking or using drugs.

We swear to ourselves that this will never happen again. But in spite of our best intentions, we find ourselves drunk or high again, caught in a cycle of using and regretting, using and regretting—the endless loop that is known as addiction. Having lost control, we feel frustrated, despondent, hopeless, even disgusted with ourselves. There is a saying in AA about being sick and tired of being sick and tired. When we reach this point, we are ready to recognize the truth.

The truth is, no matter how desperate we feel or how sincerely we believed we would "never drink like that again," we couldn't force ourselves to stop. We can't overpower an addiction. *An addiction is beyond our power to control.* Only when we admit we are powerless over how we use alcohol or drugs can we begin to be free. Only when we realize we can't quit any time we like do we finally have a chance to stop the cycle.

ARE WE REALLY POWERLESS?

The word *powerless* is a problem for many women. Many of us were taught to let something or someone else control our lives. It can be difficult to acknowledge we are powerless over our addictions because we already feel powerless in so many other areas of our lives. Admitting powerlessness may appear to be one more instance of our familiar one-down position. It seems like too much to ask of us.

Yet only when we admit our powerlessness and lack of control over our addiction can we begin to find out where we truly have power in our lives. This is the first of many paradoxes we experience in recovery.

For women, recovery is about empowerment—finding and using our true inner power. It may seem contradictory to claim our power when we've just admitted our powerlessness, but actually we are made more powerful by this admission. How can this be true? It's very simple. By admitting our powerlessness over our addiction, we are freeing ourselves to turn our attention to areas where we *do* have control. When we give up the struggle to control the things we can't control, we begin to discover our true source of power.

Questioning the idea of powerlessness doesn't mean we abandon or ignore Step One. Many women who have walked the Twelve Step path translate this Step into words that help them discover how the ideas of powerlessness and unmanageability fit their personal experience. We have the freedom to interpret this Step in whatever way helps us recognize the power of our addiction.

The idea of powerlessness made Sandy, who sought help for her destructive relationships as well as her addiction to alcohol and drugs, feel even more depressed than when she was using. It was helpful for her to use different words to think about this Step. "To say I was powerless was not good for me," she recalls. "It didn't feel right. My body responded with a drop in energy. Rather than *powerless,* I use the word *surrender*—as in surrendering to the truth. I surrender because I cannot control the amount and the way I use." For Sandy, admitting powerlessness and unmanageability was an act of surrender that began her recovery journey.

Some of us may not question our feelings about powerlessness because we have learned that others find us more attractive if we have less power. As women, we often receive messages, directly and indirectly, that we are more feminine, more acceptable, more lovable when we have little or no power. It is important that we not confuse our desire for approval with our powerlessness over our addiction. It is especially important for women to acknowledge the power of their addictions while discovering their personal power through recovery.

"As a woman, I need to claim my power," says Sandy. "I am empowered when I look inside and ask myself, 'What do I think? What do I feel? What are my options?' I start figuring out what's true for me—not whether it will please other people or make them happy. I don't want to be insensitive to others, but I also need to be more sensitive to myself."

Maria, a physician in her sixties, has given serious thought to power and powerlessness. Maria descended into full-blown alcoholism following her divorce and became sober after going through several detox programs. Because she had achieved success in a competitive profession, at first she was concerned about admitting powerlessness—it felt too much like giving up and giving in. Only after much soul-searching was she able to see powerlessness as a way to *prevent the further loss of her power.*

"Women have always been powerless," says Maria. "So admitting I'm powerless over alcohol is really a way to keep the power I do have. I'm admitting that there's something I can't control and that by trying to control it, I am going to lose even more power than I'd already lost by virtue of my being female."

Like Sandy, Maria focuses on enhancing the power she has gained through her recovery rather than thinking of herself as a powerless person. Now that she is sober, she expresses her feelings and asserts herself without agonizing about what people think of her. This, she knows, gives her a true sense of personal power. But she recognizes that this power does not mean she has control over her drinking. The drinking is out of her control.

LOOKING INSIDE

If we enter recovery for someone other than ourselves, we may not think powerlessness is the problem. Instead it probably seems as if someone else has the problem. Many of us try to get sober or stay abstinent because families or friends want us to, or because the court sent us to a recovery program. We attend meetings to please or obey someone, or maybe to reduce tension at home.

"Getting clean wasn't something I wanted to do for myself," says Elena, a cocaine abuser who started going to Narcotics Anonymous meetings because her husband, Joe, threatened to leave her. "I figured it was the only way to save my marriage. If I stopped using, Joe would stay. That was all that mattered. I went so I could keep him from leaving. It never occurred to me that I was powerless over cocaine or that I really had a problem."

Many of us enter recovery without an awareness of our inner needs and with no sense of being powerless. It may take a while to believe we are addicted or to admit that our drinking or using other drugs causes us unhappiness and conflict.

The first step in recovery is to look inside ourselves. Turning inward is the beginning of becoming more truthful with ourselves. Honesty is essential because our addictions thrive on *dis*honesty: we have become accustomed to hiding from our true feelings and values.

Most of us begin recovery without a clear sense of our inner lives or feelings. This was certainly true for me. I was overly concerned with outer appearances, so that I rarely stopped to notice my real feelings—who *I* was, what *I* really felt, wanted, and needed. Like many other women, I had numbed myself to my feelings. As I became more conscious in sobriety, I realized alcohol had helped me avoid my anxiety and fear. It kept the door to my inner self locked.

When we use and abuse substances, we lose contact with our inner selves. While our values may urge us to be responsible, creative, loving, and open, our lives are filled with dishonesty, rigidity, fear, and distrust. This split between our inner values and our outer lives causes deep pain.

As difficult as it is, we need to let ourselves admit our powerlessness and feel our discomfort. This is how we'll stop the cycle of drinking and using and open the door to our inner self.

LAYERS OF DENIAL

When we deny that something exists, we can't change it. If we deny a problem, it will remain a problem. If we insist we're not hurting, lonely, frightened, then there's no opportunity to learn how to feel better. Only when we tell ourselves the truth—risk seeing ourselves as we are now—can we begin to change.

Becoming aware of our real relationship with alcohol or another drug allows us to break through our denial. We often stay in denial because we'd rather not experience all our feelings or face the painful truth about ourselves. Our denial also protects us from the fear of facing what it means to be addicted and from the necessity of giving up our usual ways of coping with the world.

Adding to our own attempts to deny the truth of our addictions, the people around us may pressure us to deny our addictions. Sometimes it seems that our culture encourages our communities and families to pretend that women alcoholics and addicts don't exist. Because of this, we often feel we aren't taken seriously when we try to get help. People are often unwilling to listen to us because it's unpleasant to face a problem like this openly. Many of us find our drinking or other drug use overlooked, ignored, or downplayed. This cultural denial can extend to our families, who join society in looking the other way.

Shannon, sober for two years and in her early twenties, had blackouts from her drinking by the time she was thirteen. Her brother often covered for her and even diverted their parents' attention with his own acting-out behavior. Shannon's parents were unable to see the obvious signs of her alcohol abuse.

To Shannon's delight, adults bought liquor for her, bartenders didn't ask for her ID, and police officers always let her off the hook, once even taking her home rather than arresting her after she was stopped for drunk driving.

Shannon believes no one acknowledged her problem because she was attractive, young, and female. "I could raise hell and still make it all look good because nobody believed I was doing the things I was doing," she says. Her alcoholism was invisible to everyone else, so it was hard for Shannon to see the seriousness of her condition. The denial of the people around her reinforced Shannon's denial.

When we do dare openly admit we have a problem with alcohol or other drugs, we become vulnerable to criticism and rejection, adding another pressure to maintain our denial. The unfortunate truth is that our society judges women with addictions more severely than men in the same situation. Being a drunk or an addict is bad enough; being a female drunk or addict is doubly shameful. Women addicts are often stereotyped as promiscuous, slovenly, and immoral. If we have children, we are often shamed further by ourselves and others if our drinking or using interferes with our ability to care for our children.

It takes a great deal of courage to be honest with ourselves. The layers of cultural denial increase our own personal denial system, and we find it more difficult to recognize and admit that we have a problem. We may be reluctant to name our addiction or to admit we are powerless or out of control. It may seem as if we are confessing that we've done something wrong. We will not want to open the door on our inner self if that self seems "bad" or "hateful." So instead of "admitting," many of us prefer to think of "acknowledging" or "recognizing" our addictive patterns.

THE ONLY WAY OUT

Cultural messages about what it means to be a woman also strengthen our denial. As women, we are expected to direct our attention toward caring for others, not toward self-care, self-knowledge, or our own inner experience. We may believe it is selfish to focus on ourselves. We may feel we are demanding too much when we ask for what we need, set limits, or say no. If we step outside the roles expected of us, we risk being told we're not giving enough of ourselves or fulfilling our "feminine" role. All these pressures to be selfless can make it hard to look inside and see our own needs. This keeps us in denial.

If we're miserable in a relationship, we may tell ourselves, "Well, I'm not very happy, but he's really doing the best he can and he needs my support, so I shouldn't complain." Believing that it would be selfish to think about what *we* want or believing that we don't deserve anything better, many of us relieve our pain by using alcohol or other drugs. Not only do we deny our feelings, but we deny that we are addicted as well.

But as you work Step One you can start to let your real feelings come to the surface. Consider trying something new. Just for a little while, ignore the voices saying you're selfish and demanding for wanting something better for yourself. Try to ignore the possibility that someone might treat you as if you're invisible, unimportant, or shameful. Imagine yourself, instead, on the other side of the door you've kept locked by your denial. Imagine you are in a calm, quiet inner place. Imagine a still voice telling you that you deserve to be taken seriously and accepted without judgment. Imagine that you have the right to ask for and receive help—and that help comes.

In this quiet inner place you can start to trust—or just for now, *act as if* you trust—your inner self. Soon you may find that you need less denial to protect yourself. Eventually you will be comfortable with what you find and more hopeful about your life.

IS LIFE UNMANAGEABLE?

Step One asks that we first gain a better understanding of powerlessness. Then it asks us to recognize that our life is unmanageable. Many women hear the word *unmanageable* and immediately say, "Yes, that's my life!" but others aren't so certain.

Deciding whether or not life is unmanageable can be difficult for some women because we typically manage dozens of day-to-day details and take responsibility for others' needs. On the surface it may appear that we're managing reasonably well. Everything seems to be running smoothly, as long as we don't ask ourselves how we're feeling and what we really need.

Maintaining the illusion of a manageable life can prevent us from seeking the help we need. How can we have a problem if we still get the kids to school on time, balance the checkbook, do all the chores, and show up for work every day? How can life be unmanageable if it looks so orderly?

The appearance of control and order can mask an underlying fear and lack of self-acceptance that drives us to make everything on the outside look as perfect as possible. In truth, we may be attempting to maintain as much control as we can—actually *micro-managing* the lives of everyone around us—so that we can avoid feelings of emptiness, worthlessness, anxiety, even panic.

In recovery we learn how to put less energy into controlling other people and events, and we invest more energy in taking care of ourselves. We begin to see that it's not our job to manage everything around us. We *do* have a job: to take responsibility for our own well-being. When we do, we'll have more energy to express ourselves creatively and successfully.

For some of us, there's no question that our lives are unmanageable; we hardly need to be convinced that we're not in control. Many of us have lost spouses, children, jobs, and our reputation as the consequence of our drinking or drug use. We've embarrassed ourselves in public, wrecked cars, been hospitalized, gone to jail. Unmanageability, and the powerlessness that creates it, may be all too familiar to many of us.

For Ruth, there was no debate about manageability. A minister and now a recovering alcoholic, bulimic, and nicotine addict, Ruth came into AA at the age of forty after humiliating herself. She passed out on the floor at a party given in her honor. Her guests had to step over her on their way out. It was the last in a long series of progressively worse public displays of alcoholic behavior.

Ruth's admission of powerlessness and unmanageability is definite. "Nothing could have been more unmanageable than what happened at that party," she says. "It was a symbol of unmanageability. I really did feel powerless; it was so obvious that I had no control over my behavior."

Like Ruth and others, many of us directly connect unmanageability with our lack of power and control. Vivian, who became sober as a single mother with two young children, heard a woman read Step One at her first AA meeting and knew she was in the right place when she heard "unmanageable." She says, "I recognized what unmanageability meant right away. I knew I was completely unable to stop drinking."

When Vivian woke up each morning, she would start the day by telling herself that she wasn't going to drink. But soon she'd begin to think about alcohol and head for the cupboard. "And that would be it," Vivian says. "I would drink until I blacked out."

It was clear to Vivian that she couldn't manage her behavior, much less anything else. In a meeting she heard someone say, "If you were hiring someone like you to manage your life, would you continue paying her?" In other words, are you doing a satisfactory or even passable job at managing your own life? Vivian realized that she would fire herself immediately. She was so impaired by alcoholism that she couldn't take care of herself or her children. She realized her life was truly unmanageable.

LOOKING GOOD ON THE OUTSIDE

Unmanageability may be more difficult to accept when our lives look good on the outside, especially if we can compare our circumstances to someone whose life looks worse. Katy, a binge eater and alcoholic, couldn't relate to unmanageability—partly because she had accomplished many of her goals, but also because she surrounded herself with alcoholics and heroin addicts who had more serious problems. Compared to her companions' lives, her life seemed manageable.

Still, she had no trouble admitting powerlessness. For six months before she became abstinent, Katy had a daily struggle with food. She binged and cried every day, swearing off with firm resolve in the morning, and then bingeing again by three in the afternoon. She knew she was powerless; she couldn't stop.

"But viewing my life as unmanageable was very difficult because I was so successful in the world in many ways," she recalls. "I've always been an achiever; I had an intellect and was able to make things happen. So I felt I was managing pretty well."

While outward appearances may hide the turmoil underneath for some of us, there may come a time when we recognize that our public image is about to collapse. Shannon embraced unmanageability even though her external life seemed to work. She had all the trimmings—a nice apartment, a job, and friends. But secretly she knew that it all hung together by a slender thread and that her emotional life was unmanageable.

"I was suicidal. I knew it was just a matter of time and circumstance before things started to fall apart," she says. "When I went to a meeting and heard this Step, something deep inside me under-stood what it meant. I didn't really want to admit it, but I knew how serious my situation was. Unmanageability made sense to me. I thought, How in the world do these people know this? It was such a relief."

A NEW FEMININE FORM OF POWER

Because, as women, we aren't encouraged to think about our needs and traditionally do not have direct power and prestige, many of us have perfected the art of manipulation. We have learned to get our way without appearing to demand it. Because we've learned that we might be rejected and abandoned if we ask directly for what we want, some of us have found it safer and more effective to flatter, flirt, please, and play helpless.

This allows us to have some influence while still playing by societal rules. Sometimes it's been more productive to bat our eye-lashes and act seductive to get what we want rather than ask for it clearly and unambiguously. When we begin recovery, we begin to look at these indirect methods to gain power and *consider if this is the kind of power we want to keep.*

Women can have a more constructive kind of power—the power to empower ourselves and others. This new feminine form of power comes from within, from a quiet sense of inner knowing that arises when we listen to ourselves.

Despite a history of little political and social clout, women have wielded tremendous personal and psychological power by supporting the growth and talents of others. Unfortunately, this supportive, cooperative power is often taken for granted and given little value in our culture.

There is a special place where this kind of power is valued and honored: in Twelve Step recovery programs. The Twelve Steps of recovery rely on people mutually supporting each other. This is a different kind of power. It is an example of the feminine form of power at its best.

The Twelve Step emphasis on cooperative power may not seem obvious at first because the original AA literature contains many references to a very different kind of power—a style referred to as "power over." Power over is about winning and losing, control and dominance. Many women don't relate very well to this kind of power. If anything, we know what it's like to be on the receiving end of it—to be dominated by someone else.

Often in AA meetings you'll hear many "power over" references. People talk about "utter defeat," "devastating weakness," and "singlehanded combat" in their description of the battle between the drinker and the drink: "Alcohol, now become the rapacious creditor, bleeds us of all self-sufficiency and all will to resist its demands."[1] In other words, alcohol wins and the alcoholic loses.

Rather than experiencing power as a battle, women seem to more easily identify with the idea of "power *with*" or "power *to*." This is the cooperative and feminine form of power. Unlike the struggle involved in "power *over*," the idea is to share power so that we can create more of it.

Throughout the Twelve Steps there are many references to the power of working with other people to heal and prosper in a way that we could never do in isolation. This is "power with" or "power to" in action. It's a shared experience, a win-win situation.

All these ideas about power can help you begin to explore what power means to you. Where do you have power in your life? Where does that power come from? Where do you have the capacity to join with others and create a shared experience of power? Where do you have the power to make better choices for yourself?

In recovery, we develop the power of choice. When we're struggling with an addiction, our choices are very limited. The addiction decides what we'll do and where we'll go and how we'll act. By taking the First Step, we regain the power to decide for ourselves. We can choose whether we want to continue to try to control the things we can't, like our addictive cycle, or control the things we can, like our participation in recovery. By admitting our lack of control over our addictions, we empower ourselves to experience a whole new way of life.

Let powerlessness be your partner and guide you to a new experience of power. Awareness of unmanageability in your life is a sign that you are on the recovery path. Change is possible; *there is a solution.*

Step Two

*Came to believe that a Power greater
than ourselves could restore us to sanity.*

WHAT CAN WE BELIEVE IN? WHOM CAN WE TRUST?

At the beginning of the Twelve Step journey, most of us are painfully aware of our lack of trust. We're often suspicious of other people and of life in general. Life may seem painfully unfair and unpredictable. Why do bad things happen to us? Why does nothing seem to go our way? When we are trapped in addictive behavior, life presents one disappointment after another. It's no wonder we feel defensive, fearful, angry, or depressed—maybe even a little bit crazy.

Most of us start our recovery program feeling very self-protective. When we've been betrayed by other people or feel we've been cheated by life, we want to defend ourselves from further harm. Yet this desire to protect ourselves is based on the illusion of control, the same illusion that allowed us to continue our addictions, and the result is a deeper and deeper sense of isolation. The problem is that *life is more difficult and empty without someone or something to trust and believe in.*

No one wants to live with fear and distrust, but it can seem that there's no other choice. How can you let down your guard when you feel sure you will get hurt again? How can you begin to believe in a nurturing power greater than yourself? Or a life force that is good?

But what if you could trust life to support you? What if you could turn your worries over to a Higher Power? Wouldn't life be different if you didn't have to struggle by yourself?

This courage and support is exactly what Step Two offers—trust and hope that help is available. "Coming to believe" means setting aside our illusion of control. When we do, we open a place in our life that allows a guiding presence, more powerful than us, to enter. When we come to believe in "a Power greater than ourselves" we realize that we are not alone. We don't have to do it all ourselves. We can stop trying to control. When we begin to trust, we feel lighter, more at ease.

FINDING SOMETHING TO BELIEVE IN

Coming to believe doesn't happen all at once. It may take a long time for us to gradually discover all our personal beliefs and values. Knowing what we believe about *anything* can be a good start on the Twelve Step journey, because, as women, we learn to give up our inner knowing to conform to others' expectations and gain acceptance. Quite often we sacrifice some of our most important beliefs for the sake of relationships; for instance, some of us give up our religious tradition when we marry. But giving up beliefs and values can be something we do in many other ways too: it might mean we don't act on what our inner wisdom tells us is right.

Natalie, a recovering alcoholic, found herself in this situation. "The man I've been seeing asked me to marry him," says Natalie, "and I desperately want to be in a relationship. But he wants me to convert to his faith and spend a year with his religious teacher, and I'm afraid he'll leave me if I say no. Something tells me this is not my spiritual path, and I'm beginning to feel uneasy—like he's pressuring me."

In another situation, a woman stopped supporting liberal social causes when she became involved with politically conservative friends. It was puzzling: Had she become more conservative herself? Or was she unable to reconcile her liberal beliefs with her desire for these new relationships? What did she really believe?

Like these two women, we may lose touch with how we really feel about many things when we fear we will be abandoned. We get further and further away from our real beliefs when we try to please other people or avoid their rejection. In recovery we learn to listen to our inner wisdom and reacquaint ourselves with what we know to be right and true for ourselves.

SOMETIMES QUICKLY, SOMETIMES SLOWLY

The "Power greater than ourselves" is always there for us. We come to believe in and connect to a Higher Power in our own time and in our own way—sometimes quickly, sometimes slowly.

Set aside what someone in your family or love life or community might think. How do you feel about the idea of a Power greater than yourself? Do you feel comforted by this idea? Frightened? Threatened? Angry? Does it make sense to you, or does it sound a little old-fashioned, maybe too much like Sunday school? What is your personal belief?

You are not alone if you feel skeptical about a universal force or guiding spirit. That was my attitude too when I began my recovery. How could the world be so violent and terrifying if there was any intelligence guiding it? It just didn't make sense. I didn't believe there was a God: there was no Power greater than myself. God must have been invented by someone completely different from me, and this "invention" didn't fit into my life.

Like others in recovery, I did eventually come to believe in my own Higher Power. I saw this power working in other people's lives before I began to believe it for myself. I saw it most clearly in my sponsor, a woman with an inner serenity I admired. When she told me her serenity came from her belief in a Higher Power, I knew I wanted to find my own.

My belief also grew from experiencing the miraculous changes in my own life. Without my consciously willing it, my relationships began to improve, my attitude became more positive, and my "bad luck" started to change. How did these changes happen? I gradually found myself believing that there was *a life force I could learn to cooperate with* that brought about all this healthy change.

When we need a sign that a transforming power exists, we can listen to the stories that other women tell in Twelve Step meetings. In their stories, we can hear how they discovered the strength and resources to survive what they have been through and even to start a new life. We can learn that their lives, just like ours, were disrupted or nearly destroyed by their addictions—and yet in their recovery they have found *a grace that guides them through.*

How do we receive this grace? We simply come to believe. Assuming that we come to believe, whether quickly or slowly, exactly what or whom do we believe in? Where do we place our trust? What exactly is meant by "a Power greater than ourselves"?

CREATING A PERSONAL IMAGE OF GOD

"A Power greater than ourselves" may be a familiar idea because many of us are accustomed to thinking that power is outside us. We often look to the external world, and often to men, for protection and safety. Even if we don't rely on a particular man, we often find ourselves guided by institutions that are based on masculine ways of seeing and experiencing the world.

This reliance on external, masculine guidance may be particularly powerful for those of us raised with traditional Judeo-Christian religious teachings. As we begin to consider our images of a Power greater than ourselves, we may ask, If I interpret this power as a masculine, paternal, reward-and-punishment God, how will that affect my sense of personal power? How can I, as a woman, connect with this image?

The traditional Judeo-Christian God is only one image of this Power greater than ourselves. There are many others. Some women feel more comfortable using feminine, neutral, or personal images. This practice—creating our own conception of a guiding spirit—is exactly what the founders of AA intended us to do. In fact, the Big Book of Alcoholics Anonymous encourages us to create our own individual interpretation of this power.

The Big Book suggests that we choose our own conception of God,[1] making the spiritual foundation of the program accessible to people who might fear that AA is really a church or religious group. It definitely is not.

The Big Book does offer many alternate concepts of a Higher Power—The Great Reality, Creative Intelligence, Spirit of the Universe[2]—but it often reflects a traditional view of spirituality. We see many references to God as "Him"—an all-knowing superior power. We read that "He" is the "Father" and we are "His" children.

Male language and imagery might be confusing and alienating for some women whose experience of God, church, religion, Christianity, or Father wasn't affirming or supportive. For this reason, some women reject the concept of God altogether.

In a traditional interpretation of the Steps, this rejection might be considered a dangerous rebellion that leads to drinking or using. AA literature warns of the "belligerence" of the alcoholic who doesn't believe in God: "He is in a state of mind which can be described only as savage."[3]

But there can be real value for some of us to reject the idea of God as we have understood it in the past. This can be a life-affirming act if our concept of God is oppressive and punitive. By staying true to what is right for us, we may actually do better in our recovery if we forget about our old idea of God entirely.

Shirley, for instance, realized that she associated God with her father, who repeatedly beat her as a child. But she was afraid to give up the traditional concept of God because of pressure from her community. "God is what got us our civil rights," she says. "Where I come from, you don't dare say you don't believe in God. It's the lowest, most unheard-of thing you could think of." Shirley decided not to let go of the idea completely, but instead created a new understanding and image of God that worked for her—a loving and safe presence.

MALE, FEMALE, NEITHER, OR BOTH?

The Big Book's suggestion that we choose our own idea of God honors our experience. We can go beyond the images we usually hear in Twelve Step meetings and create healing, validating images for ourselves—leaving behind the God of our Fathers, if that helps. There is nothing wrong with the traditional male image of God, though, *as long as it is supportive.*

Lavonne, a crack addict who got clean when she was forced into withdrawal in jail, has a very positive image of a masculine God. After many years as a Muslim, Lavonne became a Christian in prison. Her faith is closely linked to her recovery program. "The Twelve Steps help me live a Christian life," she says. "They show me how to let God do what He needs to do in me."

Lavonne experiences Jesus as the first man who has ever unconditionally loved her. "I wanted a relationship with a Higher Power I perceived as a male who was healthy and loving," she recalls. "And I didn't have to do anything to make Him love me—didn't have to iron his shirts, cook his breakfast, or let him spend the night. I went into this relationship knowing that He loved me first."

If a masculine Higher Power doesn't bring you this same comfort, give yourself permission to picture a feminine or neutral image, if that has more meaning for you. What kind of image is right for you? You can start with one idea and change it later if you want.

Some women pray to a Mother God, a Mother/Father God, or Goddesses. Others visualize feminine images to represent spirituality, sometimes including animals or elements of nature (wind, water, flowers, earth). Still others feel most comfortable thinking of Higher Power as Mother Nature, an Inner Light, a Life Force, or other images that give special insight into our value as a woman. As you think about the nature of your Higher Power, you might also want to ask if it's higher at all. Where does the power exist for you? Outside or inside? Neither or both? Perhaps you believe in a Power inside you that is greater than your "ego" self, the self that represents your outer identity but is really only one part of you. Your deep, inner Self is the self that is greater than who you seem to be on the surface.

Maureen, whose alcoholism was so advanced that she suffered from hallucinations before finally seeking help, relies on "an internal guide and inner knowing." When she was brought to her first Twelve Step meeting, a friend warned her in advance about "fundamentalism," meaning the traditional God-talk that Maureen was sure to hear. But Maureen wasn't scared away. She was completely and utterly willing to seek sobriety.

When she heard Step Two, she immediately sought the power *within* herself. She knew that it was important to let go of her ego self on the outside and also to seek the "bigger self" inside.

"Developing a sense of self is critical to my well-being," she says. "There is a power in me that's greater than the small self I've been accustomed to; it's larger than the way I've been trained to think about who I am. It's my soul-self. In cooperating with it, I surrender to a part of me that carries wisdom and truth. It brings me back into harmony and balance with myself—that's what spirituality is for me."

THE POWER OF THE GROUP

Another way we can believe in a healing spirit is to think of it as the power of the group. Again, this idea comes from the original AA literature: "You can, if you wish, make A.A. itself your 'higher power'. Here's a very large group of people who have solved their alcohol problem. In this respect they are certainly a greater power than you. . . . Surely you can have faith in them."[4]

By looking around and seeing others who have what you want—sobriety, hope, serenity—you can trust that there is a spirit at work within the group that makes recovery possible. You can begin to depend on something or someone beyond yourself and your addiction.

For Ruth, now recovering from alcoholism, bulimia, and nicotine addiction, her experience of a Higher Power comes from her sense of being connected to others, being part of a group. In her recovery, she recognized that the Steps emphasize the word *we*, as in "We admitted we were powerless . . ."

"God is not an abstract God or a higher-up God that I find alone," Ruth explains. "To experience God, I have to have other people in my life. To me God is immersed in and generated by all of us." Her Higher Power is the energy, the spirit, working through her relationships with other people. It is not handed down from above.

"It really is *our* power—it's not mine, or yours, not theirs, but *ours,*" she says. "It's only power because it's shared. If it weren't shared, it wouldn't be there. It is in our midst, calling us into being who we are at our best."

We might come to believe in a power that is something greater than our separate selves, something that we can *participate* in. We can experience this power by entering into relationships with others. It is through this kind of connection that women often find fulfillment. In a fundamental way, women often develop their sense of self in relation to others, attending to relationships and seeking connections with others.

In our culture, the connection that women seek is often misunderstood. Because our society values self-reliance and competition, dependency is viewed with suspicion. Little distinction is made between destructive dependency—like our dependencies on alcohol, drugs, or abusive relationships—and healthy, creative patterns of dependency.

All human beings are dependent on each other, but it's the way we live out our dependency needs that makes the difference. As women, we have a natural and positive impulse to *inter*depend, to interact cooperatively and mutually with other people and our environment. If we do not find our interdependence supported elsewhere in our lives, we will find it honored in recovery.

Recovery is a community process based on the same mutual connection and support that women know so well. For centuries, we have supported each other by meeting in groups, sharing information and resources. We have gathered together to wash clothes, sew quilts, share stories over coffee, raise children, play cards, raise consciousness, exchange business contacts. Because of this tradition, we often feel very much at home in a recovery meeting.

In Twelve Step programs, we move out of isolation and gather for mutual support. For many of us, this may be an experience of grace. If we need a sign of a Higher Power, we may find it in the support we receive from the group.

COMING TO SANITY

Step Two tells us that our Higher Power or guiding spirit will "restore us to sanity." What does this mean? Does it imply we're not sane in some way? For many of us, our lives do seem to be insane. We keep repeating self-destructive patterns of drinking or using drugs. We very much want our lives to be restored to sanity. And some of us have fears about our *personal* sanity. We may be afraid that we might actually be crazy: what else could possibly explain our behavior?

Although we may have different interpretations of insanity, AA has a definition that works for many people: *insanity is doing the same thing over and over, expecting different results.*

How are we to be restored to sanity? We might read Step Two and get the idea that sanity comes from an external source. The language of this Step seems to imply that we passively wait for sanity.

But we really create our own sanity by choosing to be a recovering woman and being open to a Higher Power.

THE SAFETY OF "INSANITY"

For some of us, it's safer to believe there's something wrong with us than to be aware of the reality of our lives. This is especially true for women who have been victims of physical, emotional, and sexual abuse, either as children or adults. It can be easier to think we're the crazy ones than to acknowledge how hopeless we feel in an abusive situation.

Some of us tell ourselves that maybe we're just too sensitive, too dramatic, or too demanding. We may try to convince ourselves that things aren't really too bad or too far out of control. It can be terrifying to realize the abuse or dysfunction that surrounds us.

Eve comes from a "crazy-making" environment where she couldn't speak up for herself or express her feelings without the risk of being shamed or punished. She grew up in a family that hid its addictions and abuse behind a respectable middle-class front. No one in the family was supposed to notice that anything was wrong.

Eve couldn't disagree with her family's version of reality without provoking physical or emotional abuse. So she began to deny and doubt her own feelings and perceptions because they made it too hard for her to survive. By age fourteen she was numbing herself with alcohol, speed, cigarettes, sex, and pot.

"I couldn't trust my own intuition," she says. "If I walked into a room and sensed hostility but everyone was pretending to be the best of friends, I would feel a little nuts. I would start to believe that there was really no hostility there, that I was just making it up. Then I would wonder what was wrong with me. Had I imagined the hostility in the first place?"

Eve has gradually learned that when something feels wrong, it doesn't mean that something is wrong with her. Sometimes it's still not safe to share her feelings aloud, but she can tell the truth to herself. "I don't have to believe I'm insane just because I see things other people may not want to see," she says.

Even when our families aren't obviously abusive, they may make us wonder about our sanity. Julia, for instance, has received little support from her cynical though charming family. Julia's mother died when she was nine, but she couldn't grieve her mother's death openly, because no one in her family was allowed to feel sad. She felt so isolated, her self-esteem gradually sank lower and lower, finally leaving her depressed and suicidal.

When she began her recovery, Julia hated herself and thought life was meaningless. "That was my version of insanity," she says. "I think it's the kind of insanity that afflicts most women. And it's a total distortion of reality. I don't think I was ever really crazy, but my self-image was distorted."

For Julia sanity means self-love and self-caring. After a couple of years of sobriety, she realized her view of reality was different from her family's. Julia had always felt something was wrong with her because she took things too seriously, while to her family everything was a joke. Once she understood her outlook was a *strength,* her self-respect began to grow. "We can be made to feel we're crazy, but we can come to understand that we are not now and never were," she says today.

REAL INSANITY

Like Eve and Julia, you can think of insanity as being disconnected from your own reality. Possibly you are more concerned with the traditional definition of insanity, especially if you have a family history of mental disorders.

It's sometimes difficult to tell if a woman is mentally ill or not, particularly when alcohol or drug addiction is involved. Because society defines mental health differently for men and women, certain behaviors and psychological states of women are often considered "abnormal." It's disturbing that, historically, most patients in mental institutions have been female. Are all these women really mentally ill, or are some of them just outside the bounds of what is considered normal for men? It's impossible to tell.

The mental health field is gradually getting better at understanding women, but women addicts are still at risk for being misdiagnosed. The symptoms of addiction among women are not universally recognized in medicine and psychology, and female alcoholics or addicts are often misdiagnosed as mentally ill.

Ironically, some women actually would prefer a diagnosis of insanity. In some ways it's more acceptable to be mentally ill than to carry the shame of addiction. We can also hide behind the label of insanity, staying in denial and avoiding the issue of our addiction: why stop drinking and using if we're insane?

However, many other women have a genuine fear of crossing over a line into mental illness. Our fear of losing our sanity may be extreme and acute, especially in early recovery. Constance, who came from a family with a history of mental disorders, was terrified of descending into mental illness. When she became sober, she realized that she suffered from severe anxiety attacks, an awareness that had been concealed by her longtime use of alcohol and amphetamines.

"I had to confront that I was a very shy, socially anxious person," she recalls. "I thought I would go crazy in the first year and a half of my sobriety because I was so consumed with anxiety." For that first eighteen months, Constance was so distraught that she wouldn't sleep in a bed. Instead she slept wrapped in a quilt sitting up on a couch, rocking herself.

To get through this difficult period, Constance relied on what she learned from Step Two, that there was a power that would restore her to sanity. To her, this meant that she could rely on something other than herself to carry her through. Step Two reminded her that she was not alone. She began to hope that she could get better.

"I sometimes repeated Step Two thousands of times a day to keep from flying apart, to reassure myself that there was help for me," Constance remembers. "When I started my recovery, I was angry and cynical, and I hated God. But somehow I was able to feel this incredible atmosphere of love in the environment I was recovering in. That's how I experienced the power greater than myself. It brought me hope, which ultimately got me through the worst times."

A SENSE OF BELONGING

Coming to believe in "a Power greater than ourselves" is a significant step toward connecting with a healing energy already at work in the world. Our healing, however, does not take place if we remain passive. Instead we join with it by becoming receptive to the idea of spiritual guidance—whether that comes from a Higher Power, an Inner Knowing, or in some other form.

This healing energy, this grace, can become a guiding presence in your own life. After you've been recovering for a while, you might find yourself responding naturally to situations with confidence and strength, without any conscious effort on your part. You may wonder aloud, "Did I do that?" as you observe yourself relating to the world in new, more constructive ways.

This grace might surprise you. You might find a new job or a new home just when you lose an old one. Unexpected pleasures and helpful events may come your way without you having to make them happen. You might wonder, "Who did it?" Who, indeed. Grace is the work of a Higher Power in your life.

Even if you don't believe it yet, you can begin by being *willing* to believe in this power. If you walk in the direction of faith, you will eventually find it.

In our addictions, we were isolated and alone. Now we have an opportunity to experience belonging. We belong to a recovery community that shares the power to give and receive support. We are also part of a larger universe that supports us. With the support of this foundation, we participate in the transformative work of our own recovery.

Step Three

*Made a decision to turn our will and our lives
over to the care of God* as we understood Him.

WHEN WE ADMIT OUR POWERLESSNESS over our addiction, we learn an important truth: there are some things in our lives we simply can't control. We weren't always in control of what we did to satisfy our cravings or how we behaved on a binge. It can be a humbling and scary experience to see how little control we may have over some of our behaviors.

Besides our addictions, there are many more things we can't control. Although we may try to get things to go our way, other people continue to do what they want and situations don't always go in our favor. This can leave us feeling frustrated, angry, and resentful.

As women, we try to control in various ways. Many of us use helplessness or dishonesty or guilt to get the results we want. Or we try to "fix" or "take care of" things, even if no one needs our help. And sometimes we use our sexuality to get power over other people—either to punish or reward them. Or we may try to maintain control by bullying or threatening others into cooperating with us.

We might use these tactics deliberately, but not maliciously. When we want to control, or fix, or influence a situation, it is often because we're frightened and anxious. We may be trying to avoid feeling completely powerless. It's depressing to feel that we always have to submit to someone else's demands or that life is leading us in directions we don't want to go. The problem is that we get caught up in the struggle of trying to control things that we can't.

When we are caught in this struggle, it's like trying to carry a burden that's too heavy. All our available energy goes into balancing the weight to keep ourselves from falling over. We stagger under the weight, and we can't do anything else until we set it down and let it go.

Step Three tells us we can let go of our burden. When we let go, something or someone else can take over. Now we can be free to live with new, creative energy.

THE WISDOM TO KNOW THE DIFFERENCE

Most of us don't welcome the idea of letting go because it's frightening. Who or what will take charge of our lives if we don't? We may mistakenly believe that we can prevent more pain if we just keep holding on.

It's easy to think this way as long as we believe that we're responsible for everything. But are we? The fact is, *we can only be responsible for ourselves*—our own actions and attitudes. Everything else is beyond our control. In AA we hear the Serenity Prayer:

> *God grant me the serenity*
> *to accept the things I cannot change,*
> *courage to change the things I can,*
> *and wisdom to know the difference.*[1]

I can't count the number of times I've said the Serenity Prayer in my recovery. I say it often to help me step back from my situation and see the bigger picture. True to its name, it calms me and then helps me remember that the universe isn't always going to cooperate with my wishes and plans.

The Serenity Prayer can remind us to look for guidance from the spiritual power that we have discovered for ourselves in Step Two. Then in Step Three we decide to let this spirit or power guide life, rather than trying to control life ourselves. We simply make a decision to connect with our Higher Power.

THE PROMISE OF RELIEF

Why is giving up *trying to control* so important? Because we can't grow in our recovery if we keep trying to change things beyond our power to change. We get weighed down trying to do the impossible. This distracts us from attending to what we really can change.

Women frequently say they fear everything will fall apart if they stop trying to control. But consider this instead: *it may be that things are supposed to fall apart,* and we'll only exhaust ourselves trying to prevent that from happening. When we put ourselves in the position of holding everything together, it's like trying to stop a boulder that's rolling downhill.

For instance, if you're always the go-between in your family— listening to everyone's side of the story and trying to make sure that everyone gets along—your job will never end because there will always be some conflict in a family. If your role is to prevent conflicts from escalating, you will always be mediating and trying to keep everyone's emotions under control. No one, including you, can change or grow in this situation.

But ask yourself why it's your responsibility to manage everyone else's feelings. What would happen if you focused instead on your own emotional needs? Maybe your family would face lots of uproar and upheaval, but that's already going on under the surface. If you stop trying to "fix" the problem, it might move in a surprising new direction.

While letting go can feel terrifying, it can also offer relief and new possibilities. The lives of contemporary women are typically overburdened with responsibilities; millions of us struggle to pay the bills or have demanding jobs that require us to balance careers and families. Many of us raise children by ourselves, take care of elderly parents, and hold a family together. We may actually feel grateful to discover that it's not up to us to keep everything functioning perfectly.

Women are encouraged to worry about things. We're expected to take care of all the details so those around us are free to live their lives to the fullest. Our culture gives us permission to be worriers— to worry about the kids coming home on time, to worry about interpersonal relationships, to fret about staying in touch with family members, remembering birthdays, running a household.

But what if we trusted a Higher Power to support others as we are learning it can support us? We could probably worry less about these things and take better care of ourselves. When we let go, we can focus our energy on the areas where we do have influence and true responsibility, including our own health and well-being.

Julia first saw life's uncontrollability at age nine when her mother died. Now, facing a divorce at age fifty with a young child to raise, she's still aware that many things in life are beyond her control.

"I think probably ninety percent of life is beyond our control—the weather, other people, happenstance," she says. "I worry that things will happen to my daughter, but there's only so much I can do. I can lock the household poisons in a cabinet, but I can't control a drunk driver who runs a red light. Worrying about uncontrollable things just robs us of the time we have."

Instead of focusing on what she can't change, Julia gives her energy to the things she can change—making connections with women friends and taking better care of herself. Rather than despair over her husband, who left her for a younger woman, she seeks emotional support from other women in recovery.

By choosing to face the pain of her divorce rather than try to change it, deny it, or drink because of it, Julia opens herself to receiving care from others. Sometimes she asks herself what she did to deserve this. Realizing her husband's behavior was beyond her control, Julia lets herself grieve over the betrayal and loss. By accepting the facts of the situation without slipping into bitterness, she lets go and stays with reality. "It really does take the wisdom to know the difference between what we can and cannot change," she says.

SUBMISSION AND SURRENDER

Some women object to the language of the Third Step. Entrusting our lives "to the care of God *as we understood Him,*" may seem like giving everything away. It seems to suggest we'll be rescued by a male authority who will take care of us as long as we are well-behaved.

AA's Big Book says, "We had a new Employer. Being all powerful, He provided what we needed, if we kept close to Him and performed His work well."[2] This image of a dominating father figure is very difficult for some women to accept.

This Step may appear to imply submission. But, *there's a difference between submission and surrender.* When we submit, we give in to a force that's trying to control us. When we surrender, we let go of our need to control. *Step Three asks us to surrender, not submit.*

The idea of submissiveness can be a special concern to us, because women are traditionally expected to yield to someone else's control. We've all felt the pressure to let parents, husbands, bosses, doctors, and other authority figures make important decisions about our lives. We may even be rewarded for submissiveness—receiving praise as a good daughter, devoted wife, uncomplaining patient, or model employee.

The idea of surrender can be particularly anxiety-producing for women who have been sexually or physically abused. When this is part of our history, we usually want to maintain control because we feel vulnerable if we don't.

Maria, a physician, has been concerned about turning her will and life over to an outside power because it seems to be an act of submission. Instead, she has found a way to surrender.

"I had no problem acknowledging the need to give up control of my drinking and my attempts to control other people," she recalls. "But as a professional woman functioning in a primarily male environment, I had to fight every inch of the way. The idea of letting something else run my life was extraordinarily difficult. It seemed like giving in."

Maria came to believe her Higher Power would support her. Then she felt secure in letting go. Her solution was to think of her recovery group as her guiding spirit.

"I had to tell myself, 'I know that I can't control many aspects of my life, and trying to do so will lead me right back into drinking again. So I'm going to rely on the power of the group,'" she explains. "I still don't think of it as something that takes care of me, but the wisdom of the group helps me to surrender my desire to control."

Like Maria, we can find that it's much easier to let go and release ourselves into the stream of life if we have a sense that we will be held afloat. This is faith.

Once we feel secure enough to let go, we may occasionally need to be reassured again. This is a good time to discuss your feelings with your recovery support group. For most of us, surrender—the letting go—is a start-and-stop, two-steps-forward-one-step-back kind of process. It's not unusual to give up control, take it back, and let it go again…and again…and again.

Surrendering is like learning to balance. For a while we may tip back and forth between submission and control. Surrender is the balance point, the sanity and serenity we experience when we are secure in our Higher Power.

A TWO-WAY RELATIONSHIP

In Step Two, you begin to turn inward to find a God or Higher Power that works for you and feels safe. Think about your relationship with this healing power. Is it like a parent-child relationship? Or is the relationship more equal and interdependent?

There can be a danger, especially for women, in thinking that we'll receive good things from our Higher Power if we are well-behaved, childlike, and passive. Instead of being submissive, we can envision an interactive relationship in which we nurture our Higher Power as much as it nurtures us.

Grace, who ate compulsively for twenty years and abused alcohol, says that she enters into a mutually caring relationship with her Higher Power. "My relationship with a Higher Power is mutual—two-directional—being cared for and taking care of," she says. "When I align myself with God's will, it means that I'm being what I truly can be. And I think that's what my Higher Power *needs from me*. This is a very active process of dedicating or committing or surrendering myself to something bigger than my individual self."

For Grace this often means speaking up for herself or doing something that she's afraid of doing, which are the two things hardest for her to do. "By being willing to take action—to try something different, to risk making a mistake—I'm cooperating with this expansive power," she says. "I don't always know what's going to happen, and that was terrifying at first. I've often had to let go in the face of fear. But now I'm more comfortable with the unknown. I let life surprise me with what it will bring."

WOMEN AND WILLFULNESS

What does cooperating with our Higher Power mean? In the language of AA it means "turning our will over." But even this phrase may not be clear. How do we turn something over?

I like to think of "turning it over" as having a tight grip on something, then loosening my hold. If I have a problem I can't stop worrying about, I imagine I'm gripping it as tightly as I can. Then I let go of it—hand it over, turn it over, to my guiding spirit.

Some women in recovery use "worry stones" to remind them to let go. Whenever Frances can't stop worrying about a situation or relationship—trying to figure out how to fix it or make it go her way—she puts a stone in her pocket and carries it around with her. The stone is heavy and bulky enough that she can feel its presence weighing her down. When she's ready, she takes the stone out of her pocket and this frees her from the burden it created. "It reminds me that 'turning it over' can be as simple as that," Frances says.

Of course, simple things aren't always *easy*. This Step says we turn our will over. When we cling to our will—our fierce determination that things should always go our way—we'll always be in conflict with something.

Our willfulness keeps us pushing against, not flowing with life. If we don't give up our self-will, we can hardly give up anything else: "turning it over" becomes almost impossible.

But what is "our will" that must be turned over? The AA literature has a lot of discussions of willpower, particularly the concept of *self-will*. This is the tendency of alcoholics to use their will for selfish means. "Above everything, we alcoholics must be rid of this selfishness," warns the Big Book.[3]

Women must define willfulness and selfishness very carefully. Our task is to free ourselves of destructive *selfishness*, the self-centered focus on ourselves without regard to others. But we also want to become more *self-full*, which means establishing a deeper sense of self. Too often, we begin our recovery without a sense of self. We have lost ourselves—our real identity—in our addictions.

Rather than completely giving up our will and our self-centeredness, we can redirect our attention by looking deep inside ourselves. By doing this, we become even more self-aware, exploring our true feelings and values. By increasing our inner awareness in this way, we can create a new *consciousness* that helps us learn more about who we are and what we need.

This attention to your self may seem contrary to AA philosophy, which warns against too much self-determination. "How persistently we claim the right to decide all by ourselves just what we shall think and just how we shall act."[4] However, most women have yet to claim this right. Too many of us have spent our lives being selfless.

Lack of a sense of self, often considered by our society as a desirable trait in women, can lead us to struggle with our addictions and hinder our recovery. Without a sense of self, we cannot connect with a Power greater than ourselves, nor can we take charge of and be responsible for ourselves and determine what we can and cannot control.

In recovery we discover our right to decide for ourselves. We learn to make our own choices. We give up the willfulness and selfishness that are driven by fear and experience a fuller sense of who we are.

In Step Three, we take the opportunity to focus on ourselves—not on the outer self that relies on willfulness to get the world to obey our wishes, but on the inner self that is connected to spirit. This connection guides us to use our will in harmony with life, not against it.

WILLINGNESS

Willingness is saying yes to life. The difference between *willfulness* and *willingness* is this: willfulness is gaining power over people and situations; willingness is being receptive to new possibilities.

We are willful when we are driven by a "me first" attitude, dominating others and anything that stands in our way. When we are willing, there is a give and take between ourselves and the people around us, between ourselves and life. Willingness lets us experience the power that comes from participating in life rather than trying to control it.

Willingness helps you grow in your recovery. You'll find that the Twelve Steps repeatedly ask you to be willing—to try something new, to be open to change, to let go of the past. When you turn your will over this way, you become willing. It's an act of faith and trust: you are willing to see what happens if you stop trying to control outcomes and let life unfold.

It takes time to realize that being willing and letting go is a process that requires practice. We'll need to do it over and over again, and we don't ever get it "right," which can be frustrating if you're a perfectionist like me. For all of us, willingness comes and goes. Still, we need only a little to get ourselves back on track.

We can learn from AA's *Twelve Steps and Twelve Traditions:* "a beginning, even the smallest, is all that's needed. Once we have placed the key of willingness in the lock and have the door ever so slightly open, we find that we can always open it some more."[5] If the door swings shut, we can open it again. There are always more opportunities if we become willing.

It requires willingness to take Step Three. If you feel fearful and anxious, as if you can't possibly relax for a moment, it may be reassuring to remember that the decision you make in Step Three is not something you do once. You may need to do it many times a day at first. It is a moment-by-moment process.

It's often easier to think of a time-limited surrender, one day at a time. We learn to let go on a daily basis: just for today, for this hour, or for this minute, we choose not to drink, binge, or otherwise behave compulsively. Similarly, we can stop struggling with control, *just for today.*

You can always go back to doing it your way again in the future if you want, but see what happens if you give it up for an hour or a day. One day at a time, just do what you can.

MAKING A DECISION

The subtle secret of Step Three is that it's about *deciding* to let go. The Third Step says "we made a decision" to turn our will and our lives over to God. We decide we'll do things differently, try a different outlook. We decide to become willing, or even *willing to be willing.*

In Step Three you are free to choose. When you begin your recovery, you gain the power to make decisions for yourself rather than letting the addiction control you and how you live.

This may be a new experience for those of us who haven't had much practice in making conscious decisions for ourselves. Many of us have been taught since childhood to let others decide for us, so we may be fearful we will make mistakes or appear too pushy or demanding. We worry that if we are decisive we'll seem selfish or we'll alienate the people around us. Decisiveness may feel too risky, too likely to cause conflict and loneliness.

Ironically, we may feel relatively comfortable making decisions about our children, lovers, households, husbands, families, and work lives—decisions we make when our *role* is securely established. But we are much less likely to make confident decisions about our *real* selves, directly satisfying our own inner wants and needs.

Very few of us were taught how to do this. How do we make empowering decisions for ourselves and still maintain relationships? How can we take care of ourselves and still care for others?

We learn the answers to these questions in our recovery process. The Steps offer guidance for learning about and becoming responsible for ourselves and for connecting that newfound sense of self to a guiding spirit. At our meetings we learn from other women how they have discovered a sense of balance between self and others in their recovery. And in relationship with others in recovery, we have the opportunity to test and grow confident with our ability to make empowering decisions that support both ourselves and others.

There are many decisions we will make in Step Three. We can make a decision about how our Higher Power fits into our lives. We used to organize our lives around our substance of choice. Now we can decide to place spirituality at the center of our lives.

We can use the energy we spent on drinking, eating, or gambling to cooperate with the ebb and flow of life. We can decide to become willing to go with the tide rather than struggling against it—choosing to participate in our recovery rather than fighting it or waiting for it to happen.

Especially important, we can decide to give up knowing all the answers. Marta expresses it well: "In Step Three, I release who I thought I was and let go of that image so something else can come in. The moment of surrender is when I allow for the possibility that I can act differently, even though I don't know what I'm supposed to do. I pause and say, 'I don't know and I give up.' I know I can't go back where I was, but I don't know what's coming next. It's my Higher Power's job to supply the answers."

Marta is describing acceptance and surrender—willingness. When we make a decision to turn our will and our lives over, surrender becomes possible. We release our struggle to make things turn out a certain way. We stop fighting the things we can't fight. We trust that the universe will lead us in the right direction and give us what we need. We enter into the deepest mystery of life itself.

NOT-SO-INSTANT GRATIFICATION

Early in my recovery, my sponsor pointed out to me that I had already spent many years turning my will and life over to alcoholism. How easily I had surrendered to my compulsive drinking, making it my "Higher Power" and letting it destroy my quality of life. Now that I was recovering, I had the opportunity to surrender to a different kind of power—one that would give me a sense of well-being, self-esteem, and sanity.

Why should surrendering to a Higher Power be any more difficult than surrendering to an addiction? The biggest difficulty may be that we don't see the results as quickly. As addicts, our driving principle is instant gratification: we don't want to wait, we want it *now*. It may be frustrating to discover that the rewards of recovery often come to us gradually, and maybe even undramatically.

Because we're accustomed to an immediate payoff, we may feel uncomfortable if we don't experience instant relief. In times like this we call on our faith in a Higher Power to remind us that we don't have to know all the answers just yet. We simply trust that we will be supported and remember that life may unfold differently than we'd planned.

When we say yes to life, we surrender. Life becomes our partner, not a thing to control or be controlled by. We can relax, slow down, enjoy serenity. It may take time to adjust to the new pace of your life of sobriety. But once you do, you can make conscious decisions and embrace a Higher Power that works in your favor. Naming this power however you choose, you can cooperate with it, care for it, and learn how to surrender to its grace.

When we claim our true power, leaving behind willfulness and entering into willingness, we commit ourselves to spiritual growth. Now we seek the inner wisdom to know the difference between what we can control and what we cannot.

Step Four

Made a searching and fearless
moral inventory of ourselves.

STEP FOUR ASKS THAT WE CONTINUE our self-discovery by taking a careful and in-depth look at ourselves, particularly our behaviors, attitudes, and experiences that contributed to our compulsive behaviors. When we first encounter this Step, it may seem overwhelming; feelings of guilt, shame, confusion, and hurt are common.

When we carry intense guilt, we can hardly bear the thought of reviewing our past deeds. It may feel too painful to think about how we have hurt others and hurt ourselves. We may question the value of opening old wounds and remembering scenes we'd rather forget. Wouldn't it be better to forget the past and move on?

That was certainly my first reaction to Step Four. How could I possibly take "a searching and fearless" look at myself? Like most women in early recovery, I felt guilty and ashamed about many things in my life. I got beyond the fear and anxiety about Step Four by being gentle with myself. I gradually realized that I could take this Step in a spirit of self-acceptance.

It was a revelation to discover that Step Four wasn't just about agonizing over my past. Instead, it was about getting to know myself better. As one woman says, "If you can discover one tiny thing about yourself that gives you some insight, you've done a Fourth Step."

WHY MAKE AN INVENTORY?

Step Four offers us an opportunity for self-exploration, perhaps our first opportunity. The more we know about ourselves—our personal history, feelings, motivations, behaviors, and attitudes—the less likely we are to go back to drinking or using (or overspending, bingeing, or other compulsive behaviors). Think of this Step as turning on a light in a pitch-dark room: If you continue to walk around in the dark, you'll probably keep tripping over the furniture and bruising yourself. But when you turn on the light, you can see where you're going. In the same way, the Step Four inventory sheds light on the obstacles in your path. By taking an inventory you'll be able to see what stands in the way of your recovery.

You might also think of an inventory as a ritual housecleaning. You sort through your life, looking for the unwanted, outdated clutter that's taking up space. You decide what's worth keeping and throw the rest away. Only then can you make room for something new. When your inner house is clean and clear, a Higher Power can guide your thoughts and actions.

WHAT IS AN INVENTORY?

Basically, an inventory is a list, or description, of your personal history. Although there are many ways to approach creating an inventory, the result is an account of your life, usually written, that considers questions such as these: What have been the significant events in your life? How did you react to those events? What kinds of relationships have you had with other people? How have you behaved in your relationships? What are your innermost feelings and your basic attitudes towards life? How have you come to be the person you are today?

The goal of this self-questioning is to better understand the role that you and others have played in shaping your life. You might summarize Step Four by asking yourself these two questions: *What has contributed to how my life has evolved? How am I responsible for the way my life has evolved?* When you actively face yourself and your past, you begin to take charge of your life.

Putting your inventory in writing makes it easier to keep track of your thoughts and insights. A written inventory will also prepare you for later Steps. And writing involves you in tangible action with visible results.

For some women, this is the first Step that really makes sense because it involves an external activity. The earlier Steps are more abstract; they involve internal reflection and decision-making. With Step Four, we take out a piece of paper and start writing down our experiences—both our inner thoughts and feelings and our outer circumstances. By describing honestly what we and others have done, and how we feel about these events, we get to know ourselves.

Just as a department store records an inventory to see what's in stock, we create an inventory to see what we've got, what we're missing, and what we need to replace or remove. With this information we can see the obstacles and pitfalls in our lives and avoid or remove them before they hurt us again.

THE SEARCH FOR "DEFECTS"

Writing an inventory would probably seem less threatening if it weren't for the word *moral*. Some women react so strongly to this word that they avoid Step Four for years. One common reason is the fear of implied judgment: *Will I prove to be morally deficient?* Constance, for instance, was sober for twelve years before she started her inventory because she felt so much shame about her sexual behavior. It was too threatening to describe even to herself what she had done.

The common expectation of Step Four is that we seek out only our sins. AA literature even suggests that we use the Seven Deadly Sins (pride, greed, lust, anger, gluttony, envy, and sloth) as a guide for identifying our maladjustments, failings, and wrongs.[1] When we do this, our inventory results in a list of "character defects," traits we'd like to change, such as selfishness or dishonesty.

Natalie, a college student, wrote a traditional AA Fourth Step inventory. She was actually eager—maybe too eager—to start working on it. As the traditional AA literature recommends, she recorded all of her resentments toward other people, taking a good look at the conflict she felt in her life. With this lengthy list of grievances, she went on to the next recommendation:

> *Putting out of our minds the wrongs others had done, we resolutely looked for our own mistakes. . . . Though a situation*

had not been entirely our fault, we tried to disregard the other person involved entirely. Where were we to blame?[2]

With this in mind, Natalie set about discovering her role in these conflicts. The result was a detailed account of her many shortcomings. She concluded that her main faults were pride, anger, fearfulness, and jealousy—all of which contributed to the daily unhappiness in her life. This gave her useful information about her style of relating to other people. But knowing these "character defects" wasn't enough. She had to look deeper to find the source of these patterns.

Terms like *defects* and *morality* can often lead women in the wrong direction. Many of us focus on our failings in a way that causes us greater harm than good. Like Natalie, when we look for defects we're sure to find them—probably in abundance!—which only increases our feelings of inadequacy. We probably don't feel too great about ourselves in the first place, and we feel even worse when we focus only on our faults.

A search for defects can be beneficial if we're not accustomed to thinking of ourselves as having flaws. But as women, we are often all too ready to seek out our faults. Even if we're brash on the outside and appear self-confident, we're probably our own worst critic inside.

As women, we are conditioned to find fault with ourselves. We easily take blame for problems, especially to save a relationship or please someone else. Natalie's motivation was to do the best Fourth Step her sponsor had ever seen. But when we relentlessly search for our "defects" in this way, we only exaggerate our self-critical and self-blaming tendencies.

CREATING NEW APPROACHES
TO SELF-EXAMINATION

As more and more women search for personal meaning and relevance in the Steps, we are creating new ways of understanding and using the inventory of Step Four. These new approaches respond to our tendency to be self-critical, as well as to our fears of judgment that may inhibit a full and insightful exploration of ourselves.

Julia has taken a different approach to her inventory, finding it more useful to think about *defenses* than *defects*. She avoids the term *defects* because it reminds her of a defective car that's going to be recalled. As she says, "God only knows that women are constantly told enough about their defects of character. In this society, we're often considered defective just because we're born female!"

Too often we internalize these messages of inadequacy and inherent defect, and we believe them to be true. But the Twelve Steps can actually help us let go of these faulty beliefs about ourselves.

When she came into AA, Julia was self-protective and defensive. She didn't want to let anyone close enough to see how she really felt inside. Her defenses had built up over a lifetime, starting in childhood with the death of her mother. Julia trained herself to hide her real feelings, because her family ignored or ridiculed her when she expressed her emotions. Instead she learned to get positive attention by being smart, articulate, and independent. When Julia was a child, her self-sufficiency helped her survive and protected her from rejection. But as an adult, she became a prisoner of her self-sufficiency, isolated inside.

Julia's inventory helped her see how she keeps people at arm's length with her detached charm. She attracts people with her intelligence and outspokenness, but then holds them away when they get too close. Although she's never done a written inventory in her fifteen years of sobriety, she has talked about this pattern with other women in the program and has learned that she creates this distance because she fears rejection and abandonment. Understanding this has helped her to become more vulnerable and open.

We must be compassionate towards ourselves as we write our inventory, but we also must be willing to admit where we've been and what we've done. What are our destructive tendencies? What keeps us from having healthy relationships with other people? What kinds of things do we keep doing over and over again that we wish we could stop? How have we treated other people? How have we treated ourselves?

The key is to maintain a balanced perspective—taking responsibility without taking blame. At first, it can be frightening to think about the many things we've done while drinking or using. Admitting responsibility can seem like a forced confession of guilt. But we can learn to *name* our past actions without *judging* them, to describe matter-of-factly what our lives have been like and how we've behaved. By describing our past actions without judgment, we can begin to be honest with ourselves and heal our shame.

Sometimes we arrive at self-honesty in a roundabout way, as Katy did. Katy had a wise and wonderful sponsor who devised a creative way to ease Katy into her Fourth Step. Rather than require a traditional defect inventory, her sponsor recognized Katy's anger at, and perhaps fears about, her recovery program and guided her in another direction.

From her first day in Overeaters Anonymous, Katy detested the program and the people she met there. Her sponsor suggested she write about the people she found so offensive. Even though Katy didn't understand how this would help, she began enthusiastically writing about the awful people in her OA group. She read her voluminous descriptions aloud to her sponsor. The sponsor told Katy to circle words like *judgmental, phony, pushy,* and *obnoxious.*

She then asked Katy if she ever acted like any of the people she hated so much. In other words, did the circled words ever apply to her? "Well, sure, sometimes," Katy recalls answering. "But I'm very subtle about it and they're so much worse." Gradually, Katy came to realize that the traits she hated so much in others were really things that were true about herself. With this insight, she could identify the personality traits and patterns that were causing difficulties in her life.

THE BIGGER PICTURE

So far, you may have the impression that the only goal of the Fourth Step is to examine and name your actions and attitudes. But there's much more to it than that. When you take inventory you also have the chance to understand *why* you've behaved the way you have.

This understanding was missing from Natalie's inventory. She came up with an extensive list of what she'd done wrong, and ignored the wrongs others had done. But by quickly erasing others' wrongs from her mind, she forgot that *her behavior was often a response to her environment.*

Like many other women, Natalie was so anxious to admit her "wrongdoings," she forgot what motivated her in the first place. Why was she fearful, jealous, and angry? How did these feelings serve and protect her? Without this deeper understanding, she became very confused when she began to work on her "shortcomings" in the following Steps. She couldn't make progress until she looked inside for the source of her angry emotions and behaviors. She had skimmed over the abandonment and incest in her past because she found it too painful. Later in her recovery she was able to face the reality of her life.

When our inventories focus only on our character flaws, we're bound to miss the larger picture. In reality, we become deceptive or vengeful or arrogant or passive in response to negative past circumstances. These traits don't form in a vacuum. We develop them as reactions to real or perceived threats to our physical or emotional well-being.

Many recovering women come from environments that weren't supportive and nurturing and have suffered either blatant or hidden abuse. Recovery is the time when many women begin to heal from theses experiences of abuse. Some women seek outside professional help in addition to their Twelve Step program. Even if we have not suffered from abuse, we may have been harmed when our families or friends ignored, misunderstood, or insensitively hurt us. Many of us grew up feeling that we were not valuable and lovable, that *we just didn't belong.*

Even if we come from fairly stable families, we live in a society that considers women less important than men. In response, we may develop defenses to protect us from explicit and implicit judgment and criticism.

Protective defenses are exactly the kinds of characteristics we uncover in our Fourth Step. If in our inventories we realize that we've been manipulative, timid, vain, or defiant, we can ask ourselves, "What other options did I have? Could I really have done better, considering the circumstances?"

Again we seek to balance circumstances with responsibility. It isn't healthy for us to think of ourselves only as victims. Also, refusing to hold ourselves accountable because we've been traumatized can impede our recovery. Still, we need to acknowledge the effects that certain events have had on our lives.

When we can see the context in which our lives developed and our behavior took place, we can see that we've often done the best we could, given what we had to work with. And now that we're sober and abstinent, we can make different choices. Even if we carry the scars of a painful past, we can be more responsible for our lives today.

FEARLESSNESS

What does it mean to be fearless about our inventories? In truth, probably none of us does an inventory fearlessly. If we waited until we felt no fear, we'd probably never get started! Rather than wait for fearlessness, *we can refuse to let the fear stop us.* We can move ahead, even if it's scary, even if we feel overwhelmed or ashamed. Remember, courage doesn't mean the absence of fear, it means acting in the face of fear. And we can ask for help to get us through.

You're certainly not alone if you feel fearful about taking the Fourth Step. You may not want to remember the things you've done or experienced. If you're feeling especially fragile, you may not be ready to do Step Four until you have spent a little more time in your recovery. Or you may need to take it very slowly, bit by bit. It may take a while to get started and a while to finish.

Most women find the Fourth Step to be a gradual unfolding. Even those of us who plunge in quickly often get stuck or decide that it feels too painful. Almost all of us come up against some difficulty. As Shannon says, "I would find myself writing something and saying 'I don't want that to be true.' It was painful to recognize parts of myself that I had never really faced." When we reach this point, we find we need to stop, slow down, or just work through the tears, outrage, and discomfort.

This is also the time to turn to a Higher Power, Inner Self, or spiritual source for guidance. As we often hear in Twelve Step programs, the Steps are in a certain order for a reason. Step Three comes before Step Four because it helps to have a relationship with a spiritual guide before we begin our inventory. We can let this guidance tell us when we're ready and how to pace ourselves. If we can turn our will and our lives over to a healing power, we can turn our Fourth Step over as well.

Having a sensitive sponsor or the support of other women in the program can also make Step Four less intimidating. Gretchen had a compassionate sponsor who advised her to probe gently and take her inventory more cautiously: "My sponsor would say, 'I hear a lot of guilt here. I don't think you're ready.' And she was right. I wanted to get it over with because I felt so guilty. I was afraid of what would happen if I *didn't* do my inventory. It was really better to wait and walk through that fear."

When we're worried about the Fourth Step, it helps to remember that we don't have to do it perfectly. Most of us will do many inventories over the course of our recovery, so whatever doesn't come out in the first one is sure to surface later on. In AA they say that "more will be revealed." But because many of us are perfectionists, we feel that we've failed if we don't uncover every detail in our first inventory process.

The truth is that some of us leave out significant information the first time around. One married woman neglected to mention a small detail in her first Fourth Step: she was having an affair, even as she wrote her inventory. Another woman blocked out a memory of physically abusing her daughter years before. Both of these women were eventually able to look at these behaviors later, but in their first inventories, they just weren't ready.

How will you know if you're ready for the truth about yourself? Trust your inner voice. You'll learn what you can handle and what you can't. And you'll also begin to recognize when you're backing away from something just to make your life easier.

The temptation, of course, is to leave out the things you're most ashamed of, to gloss over the really difficult truths. And you may need to do that for now. You may need to deny the truth in order to survive; you may not be strong enough to let all denial fall away. But the truth will still be there like a pebble in your shoe. You'll find that denying or ignoring an important issue won't magically make it disappear.

Avoiding the truth can be like having an abscessed tooth and refusing to go to the dentist. For a long while you may not realize the seriousness of the problem, or you may decide that the pain of the infection is better than sitting in the dentist's chair. But eventually the pain gets to be too intense. The irony is that you will probably experience a tremendous relief when you finally have the tooth removed, and then wonder why you didn't take care of it much sooner.

As you work on your inventory, ask yourself, "What am I carrying around that I need to release? What unnecessary pain am I holding on to? What would I rather avoid knowing about myself?" The more willing you are to look at the hardest truths, the sooner you'll give yourself a chance to know and accept yourself.

WOMEN'S COMMON THEMES

Everyone in recovery—both men and women—will have similarities in their inventories. All of us are sure to be plagued by impulsiveness and resentment. And we all have an underlying fear we try to avoid by using alcohol or drugs (or sex, food, money, or unhealthy relationships).

There are also common themes women share. Certain patterns seem to spring from our desire for relationship. We may try *too* hard to connect with other people. We may end up frustrating ourselves and actually making it harder to create relationships. You may find yourself repeating some of these patterns:

PERFECTIONISM

Many women are compelled to do everything perfectly. When we get caught in perfectionism, it usually reaches into every area of our lives. We feel we must look attractive at all times, never make mistakes, and know just what to say and do under all circumstances.

A sure sign of perfectionism is the belief that your Fourth Step inventory must be flawless! Anything less than perfection and you may feel anxious and inadequate.

We're this harsh with ourselves because we're afraid that others will reject us or hurt us if we appear less than perfect. We have a difficult time believing that we're acceptable and lovable as our human, fallible selves. Ironically, when we try so hard to be perfect, we may alienate the people we want to impress.

PEOPLE-PLEASING/APPROVAL-SEEKING

Women gain deep satisfaction from relationships. But how far are you willing to go to keep a relationship? Like many other women, you may focus so much on pleasing the other person that you forget about your own needs and desires.

With some of her friends, Norma downplayed the fact that she had a college degree because she had been ridiculed as stuck-up for mentioning it. Her reaction was like that of many women who have something to be proud of: she hid her accomplishments and strengths to protect the egos of those around her. For a long while, Norma tried to mold herself into a person her friends could accept, but in her inventory she saw that she paid too high a price for this kind of people-pleasing. She eventually sought out new friends who would accept her as she was, college degree and all.

We often deny our talents and aspirations to stay close to someone else, ignoring our own dreams and pretending we don't have opinions or feelings. The motivation is to keep a relationship running smoothly. But inside we feel as if we've abandoned ourselves. We feel lonely even when surrounded by loved ones because we can't be who we really are.

DENYING ABUSE

When someone behaves abusively towards us, it can feel safer to ignore it. But how do we feel about ourselves when we deny what's really happening?

Katy's boss took credit for the work she'd done. When she complained, he reminded her that he was the authority and that she'd probably relapse into drinking and overeating if she let herself get so upset about minor things. Hurt by these insults, Katy tried to convince herself that she was just too sensitive and selfish. She tried to pinpoint which of her own character flaws were causing the problem. As her inventory evolved she saw that her real error was to make excuses for her boss and blame herself. Eventually, she stood up to him. The result was initially painful, but ultimately beneficial: her boss fired her, but she went on to get a better job.

Because of the consequences, confronting an abuser may not always be the best option. But that doesn't mean it's a good idea to deny the abuse. We can hurt ourselves more if we try to tell ourselves that the abuse doesn't really matter or that it's our fault. The key is to recognize the abusive behavior for what it is. We can then decide if we want to go a step further, as Katy did, and take a stand.

PASSIVITY

Lois found that her most self-destructive pattern was to hang back and observe her own life. She passively let other people make her

73

decisions for her. Her relationships were superficial and she didn't really seem to care if they continued or faded away.

Lois was afraid to allow herself to become attached to anyone or anything. So she never allowed herself to get involved too deeply with other people. She couldn't make decisions for herself—be active in her life—because she feared making a mistake or being disappointed.

Many of us shut down like this and retreat into fear rather than really participating in our lives. It feels safer and easier to convince ourselves that we just don't care, but it's not very rewarding. In recovery, we may start to realize how much we've missed by living our lives passively.

GUILT

For women who drink or use, guilt is probably the most familiar theme of all. Like most of us, I was convinced in early sobriety that most of the things that had gone wrong in my life were somehow my fault: I should have known better, should have controlled myself, should have done something to make everything right. I saw myself as inadequate and felt awful about myself.

Even those of us who habitually blame others probably secretly share this sense of guilt. When we feel that we are to blame, we might quickly point the finger at someone else to avoid that terrible, gnawing guilt.

You may be less guilty than you feel. Were you really able to act differently, under the circumstances? Did you really have other choices? Putting guilt in perspective—getting it down to its right size—is not an easy thing to do. But letting it continue to overwhelm you is self-destructive. If you stay in a constant state of self-blame and self-recrimination, you'll only continue to punish yourself unnecessarily.

These themes can tell us a lot about our lives, particularly if we look below the surface. There's a hidden thread running through them that I find very helpful to follow in my own recovery: much of our distress comes from the things we haven't done. As women, we often haven't told the truth about how we feel or what we think. We haven't stood up for ourselves or stayed true to our feelings. We've gone along with someone else's agenda and haven't even asked ourselves if it's what we really want. When we are unable to stay connected to our inner selves, we create anxiety and distress.

FINDING BALANCE

It is important to remember that the Fourth Step is about *balance.* Your inventory is not a cross-examination where you swear to tell the truth, the whole truth, and nothing but the truth. You want to be as truthful as you can, but you also want to give yourself the benefit of the doubt. Assume the best about yourself. Think of your inventory as a way of seeing where your life is unbalanced—how do your "defects" or "defenses" throw you off?—so that you can take steps to correct it.

In the spirit of finding balance, we need to recognize our positive attributes when making our inventories. We need to create a list of our strengths along with our limitations, asking ourselves, What do I do best? What are my successes? When have I done the right thing? What do I like about myself?

Identifying our strengths may be surprisingly harder than it sounds. Many of us find it very difficult to name our strong points. We may feel like we're boasting or exaggerating when we write them down.

Even if you feel uncomfortable, list your strengths anyway. You will learn something important about yourself in the process. What does it say about you if you can't take credit for the best things about yourself? There's something very powerful in acknowledging and taking ownership of your virtues.

Here's another surprise: many of us unexpectedly find strengths hidden in our "limitations." One woman struggled for years with her "bad temper," and then realized she could channel her passionate anger towards things that mattered, such as standing up to the school administration when it wanted to minimize a teacher's sexually inappropriate behavior. Another woman came to appreciate how her fearfulness helped her avoid bad relationships and unhealthy decisions. But first she had to recognize her fear as a guide, not as the driving force in her life. Like these two women, each of us may discover that the things we most want to throw away might actually be worth saving.

If you keep the idea of self-acceptance in mind, your Fourth Step will go more smoothly. Remember, you are getting to know yourself—finding balance between your strengths and limitations. Take your time, be gentle with yourself, don't try to do it perfectly. Above all, don't worry about whether you were "moral" or not. Let the process unfold and let your guiding spirit lead the way. You're about to learn some very important things about yourself, to see reality in a new way.

Taking an inventory can increase our self-awareness, self-honesty, and self-respect. And when we move onto the next Step, we'll have an even deeper self-acceptance no matter where we've been or what we've done.

Step Five

Admitted to God, to ourselves, and to another human being the exact nature of our wrongs.

At FIRST YOU MAY FEEL SUSPICIOUS about Step Five. You may feel consumed with fear, convinced that you'll be humiliated and rejected if anyone knows what you've done in the past. It's hard enough to look at ourselves in Step Four. Sharing our inventories with another person may seem impossible.

When I got ready to do Step Five, I worried: What will this person think of me? Will she continue to like me and want to be my sponsor? I struggled with my fear and went ahead with the Fifth Step anyway, trusting the advice of women who had been sober longer than I.

To my surprise, I felt tremendous relief when I did my Fifth Step. My sponsor accepted me just as I was, secrets and all. She didn't judge me. Instead, she listened and understood. For me, this was a giant step out of isolation and toward a sense of belonging. By receiving uncritical acceptance from another woman, I began to accept myself and let go of the guilt and remorse I'd carried for so long.

Countless other women have similar experiences with Step Five. Our shame begins to lift when we realize that someone will stand beside us *no matter what we've done.*

"ANOTHER HUMAN BEING"

We tell the truth to someone else in Step Five after having told the truth to ourselves in our Fourth Step. We can read our Fourth Step inventories aloud from beginning to end to this person, or we can summarize what we learned from doing our inventory. If this sounds too formal or structured, you can simply tell a good listener about your life.

Take special care to choose someone who understands what you're trying to accomplish and who will respect your privacy and anonymity. You'll want someone who will sit with you through your tears and pain and fear—and maybe even laughter—as you describe your life and how you've felt about it. Your listener's openness and willingness to be with you are most important. The healing happens in the telling and being heard.

You may choose to share parts of your story with different people. You might share some of your inventory with a sponsor and other parts with a therapist, minister, or friend. The important thing is to share it all—to leave nothing out—and to choose people who won't be personally hurt by anything you have to say. Your ex-husband or lover, for instance, probably isn't the best person to hear your Fifth Step!

The advantage of doing a Fifth Step with another recovering woman is that she will also have her own story to tell. This may seem an odd reason; after all, this is our time to tell our story. But an interesting thing happens when another woman tells us she's had similar experiences: we find out in a personal way that we're not unique in our pain or mistakes, that we're not the only woman who's been where we've been.

When another recovering woman hears our Fifth Step, we may learn that she was just as depressed or dishonest or abusive towards her children as we were—perhaps more so. We get a sense of perspective when another woman tells us she's done similar things. And we can feel hopeful when we see how she's changed her life.

Mary Lynn felt compelled to read her inventory to several people. She wanted to purge herself of it, get it out of her system. She felt the best way to do this was to read it to as many people as possible. But she saved a part of her inventory for one special person. She wasn't comfortable sharing her sexual story with everyone, so she read it only to Tanya. Tanya, sober for many years, had a calm wisdom about her. Mary Lynn knew Tanya had worked through a great deal of shame around her own sexual past.

With Tanya, Mary Lynn was able to recount the experiences she felt most ashamed of: picking up men in bars, engaging in sex in front of her young children, seducing a friend's husband. Hers was a long and difficult story.

Throughout Mary Lynn's story, Tanya listened intently and occasionally shared her own experience. She described how she had used her body to maintain her supply of drugs and alcohol. She had slept with countless men and submitted to whatever they wanted, including violence. In recovery, she realized that she could live a life in which alcohol and drugs had no place and could refuse to have the kind of sex she didn't want.

Even though the details of Tanya's story were different from Mary Lynn's, her experience told Mary Lynn "I've been there too." This emotional connection helped to relieve Mary Lynn's shame and guilt. Knowing that a self-confident woman like Tanya had once acted as desperately as she had helped Mary Lynn have compassion for herself. And it was a revelation to her that a woman had the power to say no. As a result of her Fifth Step, Mary Lynn had a new perspective on her past behaviors and some new options for acting differently in the future.

Not every Fifth Step involves this degree of two-way sharing. In fact, your listener may tell you very little of her own personal story. In my own Fifth Step, my sponsor listened patiently and made supportive comments as we went along, but she didn't tell me much about her own experience. Still, I felt she was with me every step of the way.

FEELINGS OF DREAD, UNWORTHINESS, OR HUMILIATION

Even if the Fifth Step sounds like a good idea, we may feel unsafe revealing so much of ourselves to someone else. There's a lot at stake when we bare our souls to another human being. Many of us are filled with doubt and dread as we approach this Step.

Ironically, most women usually feel comfortable sharing stories about their personal lives. We call up our best friends to discuss our problems or tell our therapists about our relationships and day-to-day challenges. But the Fifth Step is different. At the Fifth Step we go deeper to uncover and remember, often deeper than we've gone before.

It's possible that even our closest friends and long-time therapists don't know our most closely guarded secrets. To maintain relationships, we may have felt we needed to keep certain facts and

feelings hidden. Many of us have hidden these "secrets" from ourselves and discovered them only when we wrote an inventory.

For women who grew up in families that hid secrets from the
world, telling the truth may be terrifying. We often experience a
childlike panic when we get ready to "tell all." We're certain something terrible will happen, but we're not quite sure what.
Sometimes when we try to describe incidents of abuse in our Fifth
Step, we become so anxious that we cannot speak.

If telling your truth brings up this kind of terror, try to remind
yourself that you're no longer in danger. You can say anything in
your Fifth Step and still be safe. When you walk through your fear,
you create the possibility of experiencing relief and compassion.

Maybe you're reluctant to do a Fifth Step because you don't
think you deserve this kind of attention from another person.
Women sometimes feel as if they're being self-centered if they ask
for anything for themselves. But to continue in your recovery, you
have to ask others to listen to you, to give you time and attention,
to hear your story.

We show love and respect for ourselves when we ask others to
hear our Fifth Step. We tell ourselves we're important when we
assume we're worth others' time and attention. Even if we don't
really believe we're worth it, we can pretend—we can ask someone
to hear our Fifth Step anyway.

Traditional AA literature tells us that this Step is ego-deflating.[1]
Supposedly it's humiliating for us to go to another person to talk
about our personal lives. This may be more true for men, who are
generally uncomfortable talking about the details of their lives. But
most women have a lifetime of experience exchanging personal

stories. Any humiliation we may feel is probably mixed with fear. Even though we're accustomed to sharing, we may not feel comfortable asking someone to sit down and hear our life story. We may think we are unworthy. Paradoxically, for women, the Fifth Step can be very ego-*empowering*. It acknowledges our worth—it says we're worth being listened to.

TAKING "WRONGS" TOO LITERALLY

The Fifth Step asks us to disclose "the exact nature of our wrongs." If we take this too literally, we might assume that we should focus on our mistakes and failures. From this perspective, it is no wonder we expect to be judged and rejected in the Fifth Step.

But the Fifth Step is about openness and commitment to looking deeper into ourselves. Using words like *wrongs* and *defects* may not help us see our past or understand our present. We may hear or read those words and automatically feel guilty and become self-critical. And we hardly need more of that. As a friend of mine says, "We've had enough of the message that being born a woman is being born wrong."

Rather than thinking about right and wrong, we can think of discerning our strengths and limitations without judgment or blame. The Fifth Step is our chance to matter-of-factly describe our behavior and experience. This doesn't mean that we read our inventory unemotionally, as if it were a laundry list. In fact, there may be many tears and angry moments along the way. In my own Fifth Step, there was plenty of that, along with unexpected and very healing laughter. My sponsor was very good at showing me the absurd humor in some of my most devastating experiences.

The point is that you don't need to minimize the difficult parts, and you don't need to dramatize them. You are simply sharing your past so that you're no longer carrying it around by yourself in secrecy. Here's your chance to let it out and let it go. Now you can break the secrecy and isolation, and dare to let someone else know you. But don't make *yourself* "wrong."

Francesca, a high school senior, thinks of the Fifth Step as "getting real" with another person. For her it's about emotional honesty—being able to admit how she really feels. She's done a formal Fifth Step, sitting down with her sponsor to share her inventory. Having done a Fifth Step, she now knows how to have in-depth conversations with others. She thinks of them as spontaneous mini-Fifth Steps.

One day after an AA meeting, Francesca's friend Jill observed that Francesca had been rude to another young woman they both knew. "You really don't like her, do you?" Jill ventured. Up until that moment, Francesca hadn't realized that her feelings were so strong. In fact, she did resent the way the other young woman drew attention to herself at meetings.

At first Francesca was embarrassed that her friend could see her feelings so clearly. But once she realized that Jill was making an observation and not being critical, Francesca was able to talk about why this woman's behavior bothered her. Rather than labeling herself "wrong," Francesca used this opportunity to learn something about herself with the help of a perceptive friend.

Admitting our "wrongs" helps us uncover the reality of the past and present so that we can change. A Fifth Step is more about truth and learning than about "wrongs." If the idea of "wrongs" interferes with this opportunity to learn about ourselves, we can consider questions like the following as we get ready to tell our story to someone else:

- Where is my life out of balance?
- Where am I not living up to my potential?
- In what ways have I denied my true feelings or even acted against them?
- What patterns would I rather not repeat in the future?
- What am I responsible for and what am I not responsible for? Where am I taking on too much blame?

As in the Fourth Step, you can also give yourself permission to talk about your successes. You might find it hardest to admit your best qualities to another human being. How do you feel telling someone about your strengths? You owe it to yourself to find out. By including our successes, we disclose the exact nature of our *selves*—not just the "exact nature of our wrongs."

THE SEXUAL IDEAL

Even if we begin to think differently about our "wrongs," we may still feel there is something wrong with us when it comes to sex. And right or wrong, sex always has a special place in a Fifth Step. We're all sexual beings, and we can't fully tell our life stories without at least some discussion of our sexuality. But we may feel so uncomfortable talking about it in a straightforward manner that we scarcely know how to begin.

The AA Big Book recommends that we devote a significant part of our Fourth Step inventory to our sexual lives,[2] focusing on how we may have caused harm with our sexual activities. Yet if we follow this suggestion, we'll only get part of the story. To be sure, we may have hurt other people and ourselves with our sexual behavior—by having affairs, by withholding sex to punish or control, by acting seductively to get people to do what we want. But many of us also feel ashamed about our sex life just because we have one!

Unfortunately, society still has a double standard for sexual behavior. As a result, we carry a great deal of guilt about our sexuality. While it's acceptable for women to be more openly interested in sexuality now than it was in the past, we're still bombarded with conflicting messages. We're supposed to be sexy, but not too demanding. We should be assertive, but only at the right time. We're expected to be sexually sophisticated, but we are not supposed to be too experienced.

Most of us become very confused and anxious trying to figure out these "rules." We believe there is a sexual ideal to achieve, but how do we get it right? The ideal seems to be to fulfill someone else's fantasy. And if we do fulfill it, then perhaps we'll be loved.

Actually, a sexual ideal does exist, but you won't find it in anyone else's fantasy. The ideal lies inside of you. I found that the only way I could feel good about my sexuality was to look inside and explore what was really right for me. Talking through my sexual experiences in a Fifth Step helped me begin to sort out this ideal for myself.

The Fifth Step can provide a safe place to talk about sexual issues. In talking about sex, you may discover how far you've strayed from your inner ideal.

Sometimes we're so intent on pleasing others sexually that we lose sight of what pleases us. We may have had sex with people we didn't even like or feel attracted to, because we felt it was somehow required. We may feel attracted to women and struggle with when and how to express our feelings. Almost all of us have been concerned with our sexual desirability, hating our bodies for being too fat, too thin, too wrinkled, droopy, ugly—the list can go on and on. We may have literally sold our bodies or put ourselves into other dangerous or degrading situations in order to get our drug of choice. These are only a few examples of the sexual confusions and issues that might come up in our Fifth Step.

Constance waited until she was twelve years clean and sober before doing her Fourth and Fifth Step because she could not bear to think about her sexual past. She grew up in the 1950s, when there were "good girls" who didn't have sex and "bad girls" who did. Constance had sex with many men and women when she was drunk. She was so ashamed that she wanted to keep this part of her life a secret forever.

There is an AA saying that we're only as sick as our secrets. Like so many of us, Constance discovered that when she tried to ignore the truth it had a way of making her miserable. She was tormented for years with memories of her secret past. Finally, she realized that doing a Fourth and Fifth Step might help her let go of the past and feel more comfortable with herself. She decided she probably couldn't feel much worse than she did carrying her pain through twelve years of sobriety.

In telling her story, Constance discovered something unexpected about herself. She realized it wasn't important to her that she had broken society's rules for women's sexual behavior. Instead, she felt sad and depressed because she had violated her own internal guide, her own deepest values.

She cried, remembering how badly she had treated herself when she was drinking. She saw how little respect she had been able to show herself and was deeply aware of how she had harmed herself.

In her Fifth Step, Constance also let go of her shame about her lesbian affairs. By talking through her feelings and experiences, she realized that she had been ashamed because society told her that women shouldn't be sexual with other women. But when she realized that she didn't agree, she was able to let go of the shame. She discovered the importance of her own values.

MOTHER GUILT

Many women face another challenging topic in the Fifth Step: mothering. Like countless other women in recovery, I felt ashamed of how I treated my own children. This was by far the hardest part of my Fifth Step. How could I possibly tell someone else the ways I'd hurt my kids?

Many of us struggle with the anguish of "mother guilt." Whether we have been violent or neglectful or emotionally unavailable to our kids, we may believe that we're beyond forgiveness. All of us feel tremendous pressure to be the perfect mother, yet none of us is.

There's an almost infinite list of things we can feel guilty about as mothers. Often we've been overprotective, so fearful that something will happen to our kids that we can hardly let them out of our sight. Or maybe we've clung to our kids to avoid feeling lonely. Either way, we burden our children by expecting them to take care of our emotional needs. They can't have their own lives if we hover around them in anxiety or never let them go.

At the other extreme, we may have been indifferent toward our kids. We may have been so obsessed with drinking or using (or shopping, eating, or having sex), that we neglected our children's basic needs. Many of us are so numb that we don't realize our children might actually be in danger. We may leave them home alone when they're really too young to look after themselves. We may ignore signs of sexual abuse. We may not notice that they've become isolated because they're too embarrassed to bring their friends home. When we can't even take care of ourselves, it's impossible for us to be aware of what's really happening in our children's lives.

I was a distant stranger to my kids because I was lost in an alcoholic fog. When I became sober, it was painful to see how alienated we were from each other. I hadn't been available to them and I hardly knew them. I had to start from the beginning to build relationships with my children.

By some miracle, my neglect didn't cause my children serious physical harm. But some of us aren't so lucky. We may carelessly leave drugs out where our little ones can reach them. We may pass out on the sofa with a lighted cigarette in our hand. We may get behind the wheel when we're falling-down drunk and drive our kids all over town. In a stupor or in a hungover rage, we may strike out at them with physical or verbal abuse. Our recklessness and rampages can cause irreversible tragedies. Sometimes our children are injured or even killed in circumstances like these.

Whatever our story, it is important to remember this: We learn about parenting from our own parents. Often our parents were wounded as children and grew up with a limited ability to take care of us properly. Without good role models, we couldn't learn good parenting skills. Now we have to teach ourselves how to be parents.

Mother guilt is a heavy burden. And it may not magically lift as a result of your Fifth Step. You might always feel a pang of remorse, and maybe that's fitting. But you don't have to think of yourself as beyond redemption. Sharing your pain and regret can be a giant step toward healing. You can be accepted no matter what you've done. The more painful your story, the more you'll need to share it with a compassionate listener in the Fifth Step. This was one of the most healing parts of the Fifth Step for me, and it can be for you too.

"ADMITTED TO GOD"

Much of the power of the Fifth Step lies in our interaction with another person. The results are clear and immediate. We tell our story and see the compassion in another person's face. In the telling, our stories become real; they're more "true" having been spoken aloud to a caring listener.

But our connection with our spiritual source is an equally powerful part of the Fifth Step. By telling our truth to a Higher Power, we open ourselves to deeper communication. This may be the first time we speak directly with our spiritual source. This may be the first time we experience the loving presence of a Higher Power or the possibility of oneness with our source.

But how do we go about communicating—admitting to God the exact nature of our wrongs? This will depend on our concept of a Power greater than ourselves.

Marta, for instance, thinks of her Higher Power as a universal spirit. She perceives it as everywhere at once, inside and around her. Her God isn't one that "hears confession," so the idea of admitting something to God doesn't fit her image of what God is like. Instead, Marta thinks about this part of the Fifth Step as simply acknowledging the truth. When she's truthful with herself, she believes, it's the same as being truthful with her Higher Power.

As a Christian, Lavonne has a different orientation. She spent a long time in prayer as part of her Fifth Step, telling God just what she intended to tell her sponsor. It was important for her to spend this time in prayer and contemplation. This communication helped her sort out her thoughts and feelings and gave her a sense of completion.

One woman found her Higher Power while doing her Fifth Step. Up until the Fifth Step, Elena hadn't been able to accept the idea of a Higher Power. Her religious background left her unable to imagine a God who would love her unconditionally. But then she shared her inventory with her sponsor. To her amazement, she experienced the love and support of her sponsor as her Higher Power. The power came to her through the person-to-person connection she made in the Fifth Step.

In many ways, the Fifth Step expands Step Two, where we came to believe in a Power greater than ourselves. Both Steps bring us out of isolation. When we come to believe in this power in Step Two, we realize we're not alone. We begin to feel connected—with a Higher Power and with other people in recovery. This connection deepens in the Fifth Step. In sharing our story with a receptive listener we know we're not alone, and we may even begin to have a sense of intimacy and belonging.

This is the spirit of "admitting to God." However you choose to do it, you create a sense of connection with another and compassion for yourself. Tell your story to your God, Goddess, Universal Spirit, or Inner Guide in whatever way is comfortable for you. Let yourself experience the acceptance and compassion that are there for you.

A NEW KIND OF RELATIONSHIP

The Fifth Step offers healing. It shows us how to create a new kind of relationship with other people. We make ourselves vulnerable and open, allowing ourselves to be seen for who we really are, maybe for the first time. We experience a developing relationship built on honesty and trust. Most of us have deeply desired this kind of relationship but may not have known how to create it until now.

Now we risk being real with another person. We can see that we're worth the time and trouble. We've discovered that telling the truth doesn't always result in catastrophe and can be a great relief.

The Fifth Step also gives us a chance to have a different kind of relationship with ourselves. Even if we've done our best to be gentle in our Fourth Step inventories, we may very well come into our Fifth Step condemning ourselves. Many of us just can't seem to be compassionate with ourselves. But if we're receptive, the person who hears our Fifth Step may help us treat ourselves with more lovingkindness.

Developing this kind of self-acceptance and self-forgiveness is really an art, one you can learn. And once you do, once you practice the art of having compassion for yourself, you open yourself to one of the great promises of recovery: "We will not regret the past nor wish to shut the door on it."[3]

We won't regret the past, but we also don't want to repeat it. Because we've taken a truthful look at our past in Steps Four and Five, we can see the experiences and patterns that have hurt us and held us back. By now we probably know which patterns we most want to change. But seeing our patterns and giving them up are two very different things. In the next Step, we become ready to let go.

Step Six

*Were entirely ready to have God remove
all these defects of character.*

STEP SIX MIGHT SEEM EXTREME at first. How can we become "entirely ready" to give up all our "defects"? What does it mean to have God "remove" them? What will life be like without them?

It may sound as if Step Six is asking you to open up and let go of everything at once, and you might feel anxious about that. It may seem like more than you can do—more than you want to do. Yet Step Six asks only that you become ready.

In this Step we become willing to be open to change, willing to let go of habits or traits that cause our lives to be unbalanced. We become open to a deeper knowing and a clearer vision.

Which unhealthy behaviors do you seem to repeat over and over? Your cycle of drinking or using is a clear example: it is a pattern that you repeated even when you felt it was hurting you. And when you were ready, you let it go.

You can do the same with your other patterns. You'll know from your Fourth and Fifth Steps where you want to begin—which habitual behaviors and attitudes you'd like to be free of so that you can have better relationships with other people and with yourself.

TURNING INWARD

As in earlier Steps, we don't want to concentrate on defects and flaws so much that we become overly critical of ourselves. But we do want to be truthful about our mistakes and the hurtful or destructive ways we've behaved.

Think of Step Six this way: *What do you most want to change about yourself?* Your list of patterns might include some that many people share: excessive guilt, perfectionism, people-pleasing, blaming, self-hatred, passivity, or dishonesty. You may have been emotionally distant or shut-down, controlling, judging, or overly responsible. Maybe you want to be more assertive or self-accepting or sexually honest. Or perhaps you want to be less dependent on your family or less critical of your kids.

All of us want to change patterns that harm other people and cause us pain. But seeing our patterns and doing something about them are two very different things. Most of us discover that a pattern doesn't change just because we can see it. We also must be willing to surrender it, to become *entirely ready* to let it go. When we do, we find a Power greater than ourselves helping us.

In Step Six we prepare ourselves for change by looking at each pattern or trait and asking, What prevents me from giving up this pattern? How am I holding on to it? What do I need to do to release it? What will happen if I let it go? When we look deeper into ourselves in this way, we begin to see how we stay locked into old patterns of behaving and relating to other people.

This Step may seem baffling. There doesn't seem to be anything to do. In Steps Four and Five you wrote an inventory and told someone your story. You were doing something concrete and visible. But Step Six is an "inside job." You turn inward, examining your motives and the reasons behind your patterns.

Some women write down their insights as they work this Step; others talk to sponsors and friends or share their thoughts at meetings. And some of us don't formally "do" this Step but use the ideas to help us learn more about ourselves. As with the other Steps, each of us does whatever is most meaningful for us.

FEAR OF LETTING GO

As we work with each pattern or behavior, we may discover that giving it up is a lot like giving up alcohol, drugs, or anything else we've done compulsively. First we become aware of what we're doing; then we gradually begin to consider giving it up. Most of us know that our drinking or using is harmful to us long before we're able to stop. Fear is often the obstacle to our letting go.

I continued to drink even though I sensed I had a problem. Before I could let go, I had to live with an awareness of my problem that made me ready for change. Drinking became less and less "fun" as I continued to be aware of my negative experiences. After a while I realized that drinking was causing serious difficulties, but the idea of going without a drink terrified me. At this point, I recognized my powerlessness: I saw how little control I had over alcohol and how it ruled my life. The day finally came when I was ready to change, ready to try something—anything!—different.

Just as I was afraid of giving up alcohol, I have often been frightened and anxious about letting go of other destructive patterns. I can see now, from my own experience and from hearing the stories of other recovering women, that there are good reasons we don't want to let go.

It seems like a contradiction, but most of us hang onto the patterns and behaviors that cause us the most pain. That's because we feel safer doing what is familiar. In fact, our patterns have helped us to survive and get along in the world. They're defenses that have protected us well *when we needed protection.* For instance, rage might keep us from feeling depressed and helpless. Or if we are people-pleasers or caretakers, we may be so concerned with others that we don't ever notice how desperately unhappy we are. We create patterns like these to insulate ourselves from pain.

We will have less need for our defenses and for this kind of "protection" as we grow stronger. Our sense of security increases as we develop a supportive group of people around us and a spiritual connection with a Higher Power.

At first you will probably feel unsafe and unsure as you step outside of your old defenses. You may feel like a toddler standing up for the first time. If you feel disoriented or insecure at this stage, you're in good company. All of us have felt that way at one time or another as we learn to let go of our old, familiar ways.

STEPPING INTO THE UNKNOWN

Hannah describes herself as having been passive and accommodating—patterns that brought her security but not happiness. When she began her recovery from compulsive overeating, she started to understand why she was afraid to let go of this pattern.

Hannah's lover, Liz, was an alcoholic, and all of their friends drank heavily. Hannah didn't like this crowd, but she didn't dare tell Liz or pursue her own friendships. She began to rely on food to keep her company and numb her feelings.

When she stopped bingeing, Hannah realized that she was unhappy with Liz and afraid to stand up for herself in the relationship. In her inventory and Fifth Step, she discovered this pattern of accommodation and passivity. Time and again she would submit to the desires of others. She hardly had a life of her own.

To break this pattern, Hannah asked herself in Step Six *why* she let others dominate her. What prevented her from taking care of herself? And the answer was that *she didn't know anything else*. This role was familiar and safe. If she didn't play it, who was she? How would she feel if she asked for what she wanted? What would be Liz's reaction?

Over time, as she grew strong and secure enough to face her fear of the unknown, Hannah became more assertive and sought her own friends. Because Liz couldn't accept her new assertiveness, Hannah eventually moved out on her own.

Like Hannah, we may be so attached to our patterns and roles that we start to identify with them. They give us a sense of security. When we think about giving them up, we face a crisis: Who will we be if we don't play this role or act this way? What will happen if we change? It's disturbing to let go of our familiar patterns; they are comfortable and predictable. We know what's going to happen and what we're supposed to do. We know who we are in relation to those around us. *The alternative is to try something new without knowing what the results will be.*

For me, it felt as if there would be a terrible void—a big, black hole of nothingness—if I gave up my old patterns. It was exactly how I felt about giving up drinking. What was I going to do at a social event without a drink in my hand? How would I get from dinner to bedtime without several drinks? It would be too hard to cope with my children, my marriage, and my business. The alcohol relieved my stress and lessened my anxiety. More than anything, it filled a void in my life. How could I face the emptiness without drinking? I was sure if I let go of the alcohol, there would be nothing.

Of course, when I got sober, I discovered that I functioned better without alcohol. This awareness helped me when I ran into an emotional wall with Step Six. When I felt panicky, convinced that I'd have no sense of self if I gave up my old defenses and habits, I remembered that I had recently felt that way about giving up alcohol. I *trusted* that I would be able to go forward, even if I didn't know how to do it. This trust was based on my growing relationship with my Higher Power. I had come to believe in a Power greater than myself and had turned over to that Power those things that were beyond my control. In my struggles with Step Six I found that this same spiritual source was present to guide me through my fears of the unknown.

This is part of what Step Six means by "have God remove all these defects." A Higher Power is present to reveal the meaning of our defenses and habits. That power supports us as we change.

There has also been a very practical side to my surrender in Step

Six. With some patterns and defects I've reached a turning point that many of us reach: there have been moments when I realized that *it was more painful to stay in the old pattern than it was to risk something new and unknown.* In other words, the unknown began to look like the better alternative. At this point I could begin to let go.

AWARENESS BEFORE ACTION

Many times we may become aware of a pattern long before we're ready to let it go. This can be one of our greatest challenges.

It's common to have a love-hate relationship with our awareness. At first it can be a great relief to finally become aware of our underlying motives or patterns. It's like a light going on—that "aha!" kind of feeling. With a new awareness comes a fresh sense of hopefulness: we can change. That hope can quickly wane, however, if we realize that we're not yet ready to act on our new insight.

For instance, you might be newly aware that you have a tendency to work too much. Then, as the days go by, you watch yourself take on one more project *even though you don't want to.* Sound familiar? It's very much like watching yourself eat half a chocolate cake or snort an eighth of a gram of coke or have sex with a stranger when you swore you'd never do it again. You have the awareness, but you're not yet able to stop. It can be a painful and humbling experience.

A friend of mine once described how her infant daughter would get cranky just before she mastered a new physical ability such as sitting up or walking. Her baby went through periods of intense fussing and crying that ended suddenly once she started sitting, standing, or walking. "It seems she knows what she wants to do but she can't do it yet," my friend explained. "So she gets very frustrated. Mad as hell, really."

Like this child, we're bound to get cranky and "as mad as hell" when we know what we want to do but can't quite do it yet. It can be frustrating when we continue to work too much or tell lies or fly into a rage—after we've identified these as patterns or defects we'd like to change.

In Step Six *awareness-before-action is a natural part of the process.* In AA and other Twelve Step meetings we hear people say that we "talk the talk" before we "walk the walk." This means that we often *know* what we're supposed to do before we're actually able to *do* it.

GIFTS IN DISGUISE

Life will provide us with opportunities to experience our patterns and decide if we're ready to give them up. It's a running joke in Twelve Step circles that life doesn't bring us problems or traumas or catastrophes—it brings us "growth opportunities." These can be gifts in disguise.

Shannon, who struggled with a pattern of compulsive lying, found that going to AA meetings gave her added motivation to be dishonest. While drinking, she lied to keep herself out of trouble. In meetings, she found herself telling lies to get attention and sympathy.

Shannon eventually realized that lying was a defense against her feelings of insecurity. She felt out of her element in AA and didn't know how to impress this new group of people; so she made up stories and exaggerated the truth. When she asked herself how this pattern protected her, she saw that it gave her a sense of safety. She had created a "false self" that she believed was more acceptable to other people than her real self.

For Shannon, becoming "entirely ready" to give up lying meant risking that people wouldn't like her if she was herself. She had to be willing to risk that rejection. Over a period of several months, and many more episodes of lying and feeling terrible about it, she was able to give it up.

Shannon had to compare how she felt telling a lie and telling the truth, falling into her old behavior or trying something new. Once she got over her initial anxiety, she discovered that it was easier to be honest and to let others see her as she really was.

Monique, who compulsively pursued sexual relationships, felt that one of her biggest challenges was to stop manipulating men by behaving seductively. In her Fourth and Fifth Steps, she recognized that she most often behaved this way with older, traditional, fatherly men. As part of her recovery, Monique kept a safe distance from men like this. But one day she was assigned a new boss—an older, traditional, fatherly man! Monique had been given a perfect opportunity to work through her compulsive pattern.

To her dismay, Monique found herself playing the femme fatale around her new boss. She found that she was afraid *not* to behave seductively towards him, afraid that she would be invisible or unworthy if he didn't think she was attractive. Like many women, she believed she was valuable and worthy only if a man viewed her as a desirable sex object.

Monique didn't want to give up the seductiveness because she felt unattractive and unimportant without it. But she also didn't want to keep acting this way. For her, the key was facing her inner feeling of unworthiness. Once she became strong enough to experience that feeling rather than hide from it, she became willing and ready to let go of her seductive behavior. Then she could begin to create a sense of worth from within.

Monique and Shannon's experiences aren't unusual. In recovery we all have chances to play out our patterns and learn more about ourselves. This may not seem fair. We may begin to believe that we're doomed to repeat certain patterns forever.

If getting drawn back into your worst habits seems like a nightmare, think of it this way: *a Higher Power is giving you exactly what you need in order to let them go.*

PROGRESS NOT PERFECTION

As you work through Step Six and see exactly how ready you are to give up your patterns, keep in mind a favorite saying in AA: "We claim spiritual progress rather than spiritual perfection."[1] In other words, you can focus on your progress and accept that you are *im*perfect, *un*willing, and *not* ready.

The key to Step Six is to maintain the honesty we've been developing through all the previous Steps—and to be patient with ourselves. Many of us become angry at ourselves when we can see a pattern but can't quite seem to give it up. We're likely to shame ourselves for being imperfect. Remember that you can't force yourself to be willing, just as you couldn't force yourself to stop using. If you aren't yet willing, accept yourself. Trust that you'll be ready to let go when the time is right. Trust that a Power greater than yourself is restoring you to balance and wholeness.

Traditional AA literature urges us to strive for perfection even though we can't achieve it.[2] The founders of AA wanted to make sure that we don't let ourselves off the hook too easily. They were concerned that as alcoholics we might try for only as much improvement as we could get by with. While some people may be tempted to cut corners, many of us may go out of our way to do the most perfect Sixth Step possible, even without this extra encouragement.

The goal in Step Six is to come to a deeper knowing, to be all we can be. We can get confused reaching for perfection. We're better off if we forget about trying to do Step Six perfectly and instead allow ourselves to be gentle, trust the process, and treat ourselves with patience and respect.

BECOMING READY

Step Six may still seem mysterious, even after all this discussion. How do you do it? The simplest way is to go through your inventory of patterns and habits, concentrating on one pattern at a time, asking yourself how this pattern protects you. What do you fear will happen if you stop behaving this way? You may have an answer right away, or you may want to talk with someone or think about it for a while. You may act out the pattern a time or two, or many times, until you have insight into it. It may take a while to make sense of your actions.

Once you see what's underneath the pattern or behavior—the feeling it helps you avoid—then you can ask yourself if you're ready to face that underlying feeling. If you are, then perhaps you don't need the pattern for protection any longer. At this point, you might be ready to let it go—maybe "entirely ready."

But ready for what? Step Six says we become "entirely ready to have God remove all these defects of character." What does it mean to say that God will remove them? This may not fit some women's image of a Higher Power or Higher Self. Others have no problem thinking of a power or grace that lifts or removes defects.

In the next chapter, Step Seven, we'll talk about how these traits are "removed." For now, Step Six asks only that we become ready. We ask ourselves what we most want to change and find out how vulnerable we're willing to be. Are we ready to open up and approach life differently? Are we willing to believe that a Higher Power works with us? This is the Spirit of Step Six. It requires that we look deeper, that we be more honest and thoughtful. Step Six helps us understand ourselves in new ways and prepares us for the remaining Steps of our recovery.

Step Seven

Humbly asked Him to remove our shortcomings.

IN STEP SIX WE BECAME READY for change. In Step Seven we ask for help in making these changes. How we go about asking—through prayer, through some other kind of spiritual practice, or maybe simply by thinking it over—is up to each of us.

Just as in Step Six, our "shortcomings" probably won't be "removed" right away. The lifelong patterns and habits we most want to change may stay with us for quite a while, even when we've become ready and turned to our Higher Power for help.

You might be frustrated with this, and you may question how Step Seven works, or *if* it works at all. If you're feeling this way, it may be helpful to think of Step Seven as a way of opening yourself to change—asking for help and letting a greater power do the rest.

In Step Seven we work in partnership with our Higher Power or Higher Self to bring about change in our lives. We learn to "take action and let go of the result," to do our part and let go of the outcome.

Many of us discover that we can be ready to change, to give up our least-favorite patterns, and can sincerely ask for assistance, but that's as far as we can go on our own. The truth is that *we're not completely in charge of when and how our lives will change—on either the outside or the inside.* We can do only as much as we are able and let go of what happens next, cooperating with our Higher Self or spiritual source as best we can. Taking the Seventh Step means realizing there's only so much we can change and control by ourselves. This in itself can be a humbling realization.

You probably experienced something similar when you stopped using alcohol, drugs, food, or whatever your substance of abuse has been. Maybe you tried to stop for a while but couldn't change your behavior until, in a moment of grace, the craving was removed or you found the strength to go on without using.

In Step Seven we expect those moments of grace to help us give up our old patterns. We stay conscious and aware of our actions and ask for help letting go.

HUMILITY NOT HUMILIATION

Many women who first see the word *humbly* in Step Seven aren't sure how to react. The word *humble* usually means making ourselves "lower" or "less than," and refraining from asserting ourselves. It reminds us that we often feel pressure to be humble. We've been taught not to be too demanding or direct about what we want. If we ask for anything for ourselves, we often feel compelled to apologize. Many women are concerned that this Step asks us to be passive or apologetic.

We can learn from women like Elena that true humility means having a strong sense of who we are. She points out that Steps Four, Five, and Six prepare the path for this kind of humility by giving us a clearer vision of ourselves.

Elena explains that she too had difficulty with the idea of "humbly asking" until she realized that it simply meant asking for help. With a clearer vision of herself and the changes she wants to make, she also knows she can't make these changes alone. She knows she isn't perfect—and won't ever be—so she asks her Higher Power for guidance and support. "Humility also means I recognize a spiritual source greater than myself," she says.

In Twelve Step programs we frequently hear people talk about the difference between humility and humiliation. We know all about humiliation—the embarrassing scenes, the loss of control, the shame we feel about our behavior. We've all had times when we've wanted to hide under a rock. We've all feared—or known with horrible certainty—that someone saw exactly what we did when we were on our last binge. Or we may be thoroughly humiliated knowing the truth ourselves.

Humility is different than humiliation. It's a clear-headed perspective that doesn't minimize or avoid the facts. With humility we're able to say, "This is what I did, and it's done." We don't deny anything, but we also don't judge ourselves.

One woman says, "My mistakes are simply my mistakes; they don't *define* me anymore." This distinction is critical. When we are defined by our mistakes, we are humiliated. But when we can see them for what they are—just mistakes—then we can humbly forgive ourselves and ask for help to do things differently next time. There's a quiet, reflective self-acceptance that comes with humility.

Maureen had good friends who took her aside and explained their concept of humility to her. It's not about groveling, they told her. It is, instead, about self-knowledge, self-acceptance, and knowing your place in the universe. "I took this to mean that I could be who I am and not apologize for it," Maureen explains. "It was a profound moment when I understood what this meant—that I had a divine place in the larger scheme of things where I could just *be*."

Similarly, we hear people in recovery programs say that humility is being able to see things as they are. This means we acknowledge what we can and cannot do. I learned in Step Seven that I have responsibility for the process of change in my life, *but I'm not in control of it.* This was a humbling experience for me. Elena says that she became comfortable with the fact that she doesn't know everything there is to know, which made her feel humble and relieved at the same time. It gave her permission to be imperfect and to ask for help when she needs it.

It's important that we don't confuse being humble with being demure or reserved or unassertive. We don't want to become so concerned with being humble that we stop taking credit for the things we do well. That is not the intent of Step Seven. True humility means we have a strong sense of who we are—*we realize our limitations and acknowledge our strengths.*

A saying I taped to my refrigerator many years ago has helped me understand humility. It reads: "The true way to be humble is not to stoop until you're lower than yourself but to stand at your real height against some higher nature that will show you the smallness of your greatness." I particularly like the idea of being great and small at the same time. It's another paradox of recovery.

We stand at our full height and claim the power that we do have: *the power of choice, the power to take action and to make decisions for ourselves.* But we also put our personal power in perspective by seeing that there's a higher nature—a Power greater than ourselves—that is vaster and more powerful than our individual selves. We can think of ourselves as a brilliant star—significant, yet small compared to the endless expanse of space around us.

This is how we might think of ourselves in relation to our Higher Power. There's much that is beyond our capabilities and much we don't know, but that doesn't diminish what we know and can do. We can feel humble seeing how our strengths contribute to the whole.

A SPIRIT OF COOPERATION

Why is humility so important in Step Seven? Because without it we may come to this Step believing that all we have to do now is *will* ourselves to change. We may think that if we try hard enough, we'll rid ourselves of all those old, destructive patterns and traits that we're now ready to give up.

The truth is, we can't force ourselves to change, any more than we could force ourselves to stop using alcohol, drugs, or anything else. If it were a matter of willpower, we probably would have changed long ago. Instead, the power to change lies beyond our control. In Step Seven, we learn to attune and align ourselves with this greater power and let the changes come in their own time.

We attune ourselves by humbly asking. But humbly asking whom for what? Step Seven says that we "humbly asked Him to remove our shortcomings." What exactly does this mean?

Let's start with "Him." As we read in Steps Two and Three, some women feel comfortable with a "Him" as their Higher Power.

They have a male image of God that works for them and is affirming and reassuring. Other women don't find this to be true for them, so they think about their Higher Power in a different way.

Jackie likes to substitute "Her" for "Him" in Step Seven. Although she doesn't believe God is either male or female, she uses feminine language because it makes her feel *included*. "When I say 'Her,' I experience what it feels like to associate God with feminine power," she says. When she identifies with this spiritual force, she feels able to cooperate with it.

You can substitute whatever words support you in this Step. Maureen, for example, asks for wisdom and clarity rather than for something to be removed. She asks the Great Spirit to show her how she can be her most magnificent self. Approaching Step Seven in this way, she acknowledges her place in the universe while asking for guidance in making the most of her abilities. Her Higher Power isn't a "He" or a "She," but a beneficent spirit whom she trusts and seeks to honor by being her true self.

TO EACH HER OWN

Your interpretation of Step Seven will be as individual as you are. In finding the way that's right for you, you may want to consider some of the following possibilities. While several of the examples below include prayer, remember that the Seventh Step does not require prayer. You can go about it any way you choose; it depends entirely on how you communicate with your Higher Power.

THE SEVENTH STEP PRAYER

Lavonne believes in a divine grace that lifts her destructive habits just as it lifted her craving for crack cocaine. She prays for God—in her case a male, Christian God and the first male she feels has given her unconditional love—to help her find release from the other obstacles that cause her difficulty.

Lavonne uses the Seventh Step prayer from the AA Big Book when working Step Seven. The prayer reads:

> *My Creator, I am now willing that you should have all of me, good and bad. I pray that you now remove from me every single defect of character which stands in the way of my usefulness to you and my fellows. Grant me strength, as I go out from here, to do your bidding.*[1]

She finds comfort in this prayer; it helps her feel open and willing to experience whatever life brings. It affirms that God will accept her and offer her support in whatever comes next.

Some women feel uncomfortable with the wording of this prayer and prefer to use words that describe a more active and equal relationship with a Higher Power. Still, this prayer can be a useful framework for creating our own prayers.

The spirit of the AA Seventh Step prayer is, "Here I am, just as I am, in all my strengths and limitations. I'm ready and willing to change my old patterns when the time is right. I've done the footwork, and now I need your help to live differently. What can I do now to cooperate with life and be the best I can be?" You may want to use words like these, or any others you like, to create a version of this prayer for yourself.

Step Seven helps Natalie stop struggling with the things she can't change, including herself. To practice this Step, she uses the Serenity Prayer:

> *God grant me the serenity*
> *to accept the things I cannot change,*
> *courage to change the things I can,*
> *and wisdom to know the difference.*[2]

Natalie doesn't direct this prayer to "God," because she thinks of her Higher Power as an "inner knowing," but says the Serenity Prayer aloud as an affirmation. It gives her a sense of humility, reminding her that there's only so much she can control.

Natalie has discovered that her most harmful patterns—her rage and jealousy and paralyzing fear—have gradually shifted over time. She's noticed, for instance, that she doesn't automatically fly into a rage when another driver cuts her off on the freeway. At first she tried to force herself to stop reacting angrily but only found herself becoming more furious. She soon realized that she had gone as far as she could in changing this pattern herself. It was time to ask for help.

"Saying the Serenity Prayer helps me remember that I can't do it all myself," explains Natalie. "It reminds me that things don't always have to go my way, on my time schedule. At the same time, it reminds me to accept myself no matter where I am."

Because she's been willing and able to trust her inner knowing, Natalie has learned to respond to things in a different way. She's found she intuitively knows how to handle situations that used to baffle her—one of AA's promises.[3] When we see ourselves responding differently to situations that once set our destructive behaviors in motion, we can be sure that our old patterns are being replaced by new ones.

Steps Three and Seven both involve giving up trying to control things that are beyond our capacity to control. In Step Three we made a general commitment to turn our will and our lives over to a Power greater than ourselves. Now in Step Seven we turn *ourselves* over and let our healing power do the rest.

CREATING A GOD BOX

One popular way of doing Step Seven is to use a "God box" or "God can" in a ritual or ceremony that makes this Step more immediate. Some women designate a special container—a shoe box, a jewelry box, a decorated coffee can—as a place to put the things they want to turn over to their Higher Power. When they're ready to let go of a pattern, they write a description of it on a piece of paper and place the paper in their God box as a symbolic way of giving it up. Once it's in the box, it's in their Higher Power's care. If they want to take control again, they take the paper out of the box.

There's something reassuring about the ritual of putting your pattern—your dishonesty or people-pleasing or pessimism or whatever—in a box and shutting the lid. You can also include the names of people, places, and things you've been trying to control. When you place them in a box, all these things go out of your hands, and you can let them be.

You don't have to call it a God box if "God" isn't the name you give your guiding spirit. Call the box whatever you like, or make up another practice that helps you visualize letting go. Some women write their patterns on paper, seal them in an envelope, and mail them to their Goddess or Inner Self or Universal Spirit, making up a nonsense address, or mail them to their sponsors. One group of women took little scraps of paper on which they described their undesirable patterns and burned them in a bonfire at the beach. Be creative. It's the process that matters.

BUILDING A COLLABORATION

My friend Grace has trouble with the phrase "humbly asked Him to remove our shortcomings" because it sounds too passive. It gives her the impression that she'll be made pure and perfect if she asks nicely and catches God in the right mood. For Grace, this doesn't ring true. "I believe that I don't ask my Higher Power to do anything *for* me," she says. "Instead, I ask my Higher Power to work *with* me. I do my part and God does Hers."

Grace assumes an active, relational role in Step Seven. She enters into a dialogue with her Higher Power by saying, "I'm ready and I need your help. Show me where to go from here." She imagines a two-way partnership based on her willingness to be truthful about herself and to be open to the unknown. At the same time, she believes that she gives her Higher Power a gift by aligning herself with it. Her cooperation actually empowers the Power.

Step Seven is a collaboration. It isn't like dropping off your car at the mechanic's shop and saying, "It's all yours. Looks like the brakes and transmission need major work. When can you get it back to me?" Instead, it's more like performing a duet. Your Higher Power plays the melody line and you play the harmony. In this way you and your Higher Power create the music together.

The result is different if we insist on playing solo. Without our cooperation, life will continue to play the melody, but we may find ourselves out of sync and off-key. This is what we did when we compulsively pursued drugs, sex, relationships, or food with little awareness of how our actions made our lives more difficult. In a new spirit of cooperation, we can listen for life's melody and harmonize with it.

A WORD ABOUT "SHORTCOMINGS"

When we think of ourselves as having "shortcomings," we may focus so intently on what's wrong that we miss the true point. In this Step especially, we work in partnership with a Power greater than ourselves, which does *not* require that we put ourselves in a one-down position by focusing on our flaws. Instead, we humbly present ourselves to our Higher Power *just as we are* and look for guidance in moving on.

Remember too that "defects" or "shortcomings" may have benefits that reveal themselves over time. Be careful about trying to "remove" anything entirely. There may be hidden strengths in the patterns that seem most troublesome.

Perhaps one of your most harmful patterns is caretaking. You may have a difficult time letting anyone do anything without your help. You may become overinvolved in other people's lives, worrying about them so much that you're hardly aware of your own needs. You now realize that your life will be saner and your relationships healthier if you let other people live their own lives, while you live yours. You've identified this as a pattern you'd like to release.

But before you get ready to give up caretaking, turn some of that energy toward yourself. If you're focused on caring for others, you probably don't take very good care of yourself. You may find that you need the attention you've been lavishing on everyone else. See if there's a way to turn your caretaking into something beneficial for yourself.

Here's another example: Like many women, you may find yourself almost paralyzed by your perfectionism. You're in a constant state of anxiety because everything has to be just so. You can't have friends over for dinner without fretting about what they'll think of the food or your housekeeping, or wondering if they'll approve of the way you've decorated your home. Is there just one more last-minute thing you could do to create a better impression? Despite your best efforts, there's always one more thing you could do to get closer to perfection.

If this describes your approach to life, this is probably a pattern you'll be happy to give up. An obsession with perfection can make you feel crazy and depressed. But before you give up perfectionism altogether, consider how it might benefit you. If you're perfectionistic, you probably have a keen attention to detail and a desire for quality and excellence that serves you well in other areas of your life.

In your work, for instance, you may be rewarded for your perfectionistic tendencies. In your personal life this pattern may help you insist that you don't settle for second best. The key is to let perfectionism help you instead of hinder you. Rather than thinking of it as a weakness, think of it as the strength and dedication to provide the best for yourself.

I had a similar experience with workaholism. At times I have let my work consume me, to the detriment of my relationships with the people I love. When I saw how compulsive I was about work, how I was afraid *not* to work as much as I did, I began to wonder if I should change. Maybe I should take a more routine job or do less demanding work. In other words, I thought the solution was to go to the opposite extreme.

But when I looked inward to find my values and source of satisfaction, I affirmed my passion and commitment for what I do. I also recognized my capacity to go too far. For me, giving up my workaholic pattern meant striking a balance—doing fewer projects and saying no to some things. I became willing and ready to let go of the piece of the pattern that was interfering with my life. But I realized I could keep the passion and commitment. I could continue to do work that I love.

In the same way you may find that your "liabilities" are also your assets. There may not be something worth keeping in each of your patterns, but you can explore the possibility. If a shortcoming is in fact a shortcoming, think of it as falling short of your potential. Look at your troublesome habits and behaviors and begin to see them as areas for personal growth. How can a pattern work *for* you?

ACCEPTANCE AND SECURITY

At Step Seven we come to acceptance. Through the last several Steps we've been developing a greater awareness of the patterns that keep us from a fulfilling life. But for all our awareness, we still may not accept ourselves. Step Seven gives us the opportunity to move from self-awareness to self-acceptance.

Acceptance is the key to change. Another paradox I have learned in recovery is that when I accept myself *just as I am,* I can change. If we're preoccupied with criticizing and finding fault with ourselves, we'll probably stay stuck in our old patterns and routines.

When we "humbly" ask in Step Seven, we are practicing self-acceptance and surrender. We say, "I accept that I'm not perfect, I don't know it all, and I'm not the only one in charge of the process of change. But I'm willing to contribute what I can, and I'm ready for whatever comes next." When we ask, we acknowledge our rightful place in the universe—both our greatness and our smallness in the vastly larger constellation of life.

We take Step Seven privately, with our spiritual source. With the HOW of recovery—Honesty, Openness, and Willingness—we open ourselves to change and let a Higher Power do the rest. Many of us find that we now feel more confident relying on a Power greater than ourselves. And with the gift of self-acceptance and security, we're ready for Step Eight, ready to carry what we've learned in the first seven Steps into all other relationships in our lives.

Step Eight

Made a list of all persons we had harmed,
and became willing to make amends to them all.

STEP EIGHT PREPARES US for a new way of relating to the world. By learning more about ourselves at each Step, we become ready to clear away the past and form honest and open relationships.

In Step Five we shared our inventories with another human being and were compassionately accepted. In Step Six we became open to a deeper knowing and clearer vision. And in Step Seven we asked our Higher Power for help, realizing that we couldn't change alone. With these experiences supporting us, we can expand even further—bringing a spirit of openness and truthfulness to all our relationships.

UNFINISHED BUSINESS

In Step Eight we decide which of our relationships need the most attention and we list them. Just as in earlier Steps we looked to see where our personal lives were out of balance, we now look for imbalances in our relationships—with family, friends, partners, ex-partners, neighbors, employers, co-workers, ministers, schools, government agencies, car dealers, repairmen, anyone.

The *Twelve Steps and Twelve Traditions* of AA describes Step Eight as the beginning of "the best possible relations with every human being we know."[1] To begin this step, we focus on the instances where we clearly caused harm.

Where is there ongoing bitterness, animosity, fear, or hostility in our relationships? Whom do we resent or avoid? Whom have we embarrassed, threatened, or frightened? Where have we purposely or negligently made someone unhappy? These questions can lead us to explore the harm we may have caused others in the past.

But as we continue to work this Step, we realize that "harm" has other meanings as well. We might want to consider relationships that feel unresolved—whether we believe we've harmed someone or not. Is there unfinished business to attend to? Which people do we want to relate to in a different way? Do we owe amends or an apology to certain people, or do we simply need to make peace or make things right with another person? We can look at where we've caused harm, as well as where we need to clear the air and create a healthier relationship.

Sometimes making amends simply involves giving someone more respect and honesty. With this in mind, we can *make a list of all the people we'd like to be truthful with*. This could be our list of amends.

You may also want to consider other possibilities. For instance, does your life revolve entirely around a particular relationship? Have you been too involved in someone else's life? Are you unhappy with someone but afraid to tell that person? Are there relationships you try to control indirectly? In which relationships are you unable to be honest and open? Where are you harming *yourself?*

These questions all add up to one pivotal question we must ask at Step Eight: *In which relationships am I not being true to myself?* Using an approach like this is in the spirit of creating "the best possible relations." When we approach our relationships differently in the present, we become free of the past.

THE SPECTRUM OF HARMS

Unfortunately, we *do* hurt people when we're drinking (or using drugs or overspending or bingeing). When an addiction is at the center of our lives, other people suffer.

There are countless ways we may have hurt other people. In our desire for more sex, alcohol, love, pills, or food, we're liable to do just about anything to maintain our supply—and that may include lying, stealing, cheating, and being blatantly irresponsible and unreliable. Sometimes we resort to physical and verbal abuse when we're hungover, strung out, or just plain frustrated that we're not getting what we want. All these behaviors will be harmful to anyone who's on the receiving end.

Francesca found it easy to understand what Step Eight meant by "harmed." She could readily see how she had harmed her family with her alcoholic behavior. When she read through the Steps for the first time in the earliest months of her sobriety, this Step made the most sense.

Francesca recalled many scenes that had humiliated and frightened her family members. She had embarrassed her mother by showing up drunk at a neighborhood Cinco de Mayo celebration. On another occasion, she drank herself to unconsciousness, frightening her sister who was unable to wake her up. When Francesca recalled these incidents, she recognized who to list in her Eighth Step.

Like Francesca, we want to acknowledge the pain that has resulted, but we also want to be aware of other ways in which our relationships become unbalanced. Some of our patterns may be more subtle than these obviously destructive behaviors, but the results are equally harmful.

OVERRESPONSIBILITY

When we take care of everything for everyone, we don't give other people the opportunity to make their own decisions or mistakes. This is particularly harmful to children, who learn and grow when they have the chance to take responsibility for themselves. The adults around us also suffer when we try to take charge of everything. Our desire for control can create power struggles and leave other people feeling incompetent and unappreciated. It's as if we assume they can't take care of themselves—or at least not as well as we can.

Annemarie, recovering from anorexia, was visiting her brother Charles one holiday weekend and decided to "help" him by balancing his checkbook—without asking his permission. When she told him about it, Charles became furious, saying that it was none of her business and an invasion of his privacy. At first Annemarie couldn't see why Charles was offended, but she eventually understood his point of view.

As she considered this relationship, Annemarie saw that Charles's finances were not her problem and that her behavior had only alienated him. While presuming to act in his best interests, she was easing her own anxiety over his finances and intruding where she didn't belong. She looked to see where else this pattern of over-responsibility appeared in her life. This helped her decide who else to place on her amends list.

PASSIVITY

Lois assumed a passive role in her relationships. Whatever anyone else wanted was fine with her. She wasn't able to make decisions for herself or actively participate in her life.

Her husband, for instance, decided where they would live, how they would spend money, where they would go on vacation, and when the relatives would visit. At first he enjoyed the decision-making power, but he grew tired of it when he realized he didn't want a submissive life partner.

Lois became even more passive as her drinking progressed, placing an unfair burden on her friends and family. They became resentful because she refused to take responsibility for herself.

Our loved ones are sure to feel frustrated and angry when we expect them to be our caretakers and decision-makers. We harm them by thrusting too much responsibility into their hands.

EMOTIONAL ABSENCE

When we withdraw emotionally from the people around us, we force them to guess at our feelings, wants, and needs. Our spouses, children, and family members may try to please us and draw us out, only to receive our indifference or disapproval in return. If we've held people at arm's length in this way, they've probably felt rejected and hurt, wondering what they've done to drive us away.

My own children felt that I was punishing them because I was remote and unresponsive. They wondered what they had done wrong, and this hurt their self-esteem. They blamed themselves for my distance and were harmed by my lack of response.

EMOTIONAL DISHONESTY

Honesty is often the most difficult issue in our relationships. Because we're eager to please and often want to keep a relationship going, we may become skillful at hiding our real feelings. We can be reluctant to talk about things that trouble us, putting on a false smile or pretending that everything is okay when we're actually furious or hurt.

Emotional dishonesty is different than emotional absence. When we're absent, we're indifferent to or uninterested in the concerns of people around us. When we're emotionally dishonest, we may show interest but carefully control which emotions we reveal and how we show them.

Ginger, a compulsive shopper, is unable to show her true feelings in her relationship with her sixteen-year-old daughter, Robin. Ginger is angry because Robin is cutting school, shoplifting, and lying about her activities, but Ginger is terrified of losing Robin if she is honest about her feelings. She has set a few limits, but Robin has threatened to run off with her boyfriend.

Ginger now tries to appear to be a permissive mom, making no attempt to set limits with her daughter. But Ginger has forced her anger and frustration underground in her effort to minimize conflict. She tries to convince herself she doesn't feel the anger. As a result she is anxious and depressed.

You may have told yourself similar stories. Maybe you've convinced yourself it's no big deal that your mother constantly criticizes your appearance or that one of your closest friends shares private information about you with other people. You try to ignore these incidents and never say a word to either your mother or your friend. But your feelings gnaw away at you nonetheless, creating strain in these relationships.

Where's the harm in these lies of omission? How does it hurt other people when we don't let them see our disappointment, fear, or anger? What happens in our relationships when we don't speak up for ourselves? We give people the mistaken impression that they're involved with us, but we're hiding our true self far below the surface. When we conceal ourselves, our friends and family don't get the opportunity to have a real relationship with us—as we really are. It can be unfair to both ourselves and others when we censor our true feelings and pretend to be someone we're not.

And dishonesty invites dishonesty in return. It's hard for one person to be real in a relationship when the other is trying to avoid conflict at all costs. Our emotional dishonesty creates an atmosphere of mistrust and confusion that is unhealthy for everyone concerned.

A common thread runs through all these "harms": we have the illusion of control over our relationships. We use these behaviors to influence situations to our advantage, and in the process we hurt others and ourselves by sabotaging the opportunity for honest relationships.

THE URGE TO APOLOGIZE

Now that we have a sense of the kinds of harm we may have caused, we can set about creating our list. But we must take care. Women, especially, may be inclined to go overboard in Step Eight.

When Eve wrote her first list of amends, it had more than 120 names on it. She was ready to take responsibility for everything—every strain and unhappiness in each of her relationships. Eve is a perfect example of how far women can go to take the blame for any and all relationship difficulties.

In an AA meeting, Eve shared—with some pride—the length and thoroughness of her Eighth Step list. When the meeting was over, an older woman took her aside and suggested that her list was probably too long. "You know who you've *really* harmed," she said. "Probably not a hundred people." At first Eve wanted to ignore this woman's observation, but the truth soon became clear.

"She was right. My next list was much shorter—just a few significant people," says Eve. "I realized that a long list distracted me from the most difficult and painful relationships, and the true amends I had to make."

When we are concerned with writing the most complete amends list in the history of recovery, we risk diluting the power of this Step. When we feel we have to apologize for everything, we can't commit ourselves to the relationships that most need our attention.

How ready and willing women are to apologize! Step Eight is sure to trigger any apologetic tendencies we might have. We may owe legitimate apologies to certain people, but before listing a name, we need to consider this: What's my motivation for apologizing? Was I in the wrong and now want to set it right? Or do I have a different motive?

Maybe we apologize thinking we don't have to change our behavior. One woman called her therapist to say, "My sponsor says I owe you amends because I owe you money. So I'm sorry I haven't paid you." And then she never sent the money! Saying "I'm sorry" isn't the point. Being willing to make amends means being ready to do whatever it takes to make things right.

We often hope our apology will reduce the anxiety and conflict in a relationship. We believe that if we say we're sorry or let the other person be right, the relationship can go on with little disturbance.

As with Ginger, *the disturbance lives inside of us* until we find a way to honor our feelings. Maybe the surface of the relationship seems smooth, but inner turmoil is the price we pay for emotional dishonesty and for carrying too much responsibility.

SHARED RESPONSIBILITY

In the Eighth Step *it's essential that women hold others accountable for their actions too.* AA literature cautions against pointing a finger at other people or dwelling on the wrongs they've done us.[2] But this doesn't mean we want to forget completely what others have done. We want to remember and clearly name the events of the past.

As my friend Ruth points out, we have *shared* responsibility for the harm that occurs in a relationship. In her view, we do the

Eighth Step by taking responsibility for our part *without minimizing the role that someone else has played.* With this in mind, we can keep a clear perspective on the Eighth Step.

When we recognize our accountability, we may tend to forget or minimize the other person's responsibility. Or we may think we provoked or caused someone else's violent or hurtful behavior. The key is truthfulness—about each person's part in the relationship. When we are honest, we clear the way for our inner knowing to show us where an apology or amend is due.

Elena's sponsor went through her list of amends with her and helped her see where she *didn't* owe amends. There were people on the list who had seriously harmed Elena—betraying her and verbally and physically abusing her—but *Elena* felt responsible for what happened. She believed she had somehow caused the abuse.

"My sponsor pointed out that I had been treated badly and didn't deserve the treatment I received," says Elena. "It was healing for me to let go of feeling responsible for the way certain people had treated me."

Before we take all the blame, we need to slow down and ask, What part did I play in this difficult relationship? What part did the other person play? Like Elena, we might find that someone else is responsible, or that some of the responsibility is ours and some theirs. We can stop trying to figure out how we caused the relationship to go wrong. In some cases, "making things right" may mean letting go. It may be time to stop trying to "fix" the relationship and acknowledge the pain or difficulty.

PUTTING OURSELVES ON THE LIST

It's often said in recovery circles that we should put *ourselves* on our list of amends. We have undoubtedly hurt ourselves along the way—probably more deeply than we realize.

We have harmed ourselves with our drinking or using. When we're out of control, we violate our values and place ourselves in dangerous or harmful situations. We do things we never wanted or intended to do. When we treat ourselves badly, we begin to believe we don't deserve better.

You may recall Constance, who was so ashamed of her sexual behavior she couldn't do a Fourth and Fifth Step until she'd been sober for many years. Hannah felt equally self-critical because her compulsive eating had numbed her to the unpleasant realities of her relationship with an alcoholic partner. Lavonne supported her crack habit with prostitution and suffered deep humiliation when her children were taken away. In every case there was a painful price. All of these women had damaged their self-esteem. They felt ashamed and degraded by their out-of-control behavior.

Healthy relationships are impossible when we are drinking, using, or otherwise behaving compulsively. And when we're alienated in our relationships, we feel worthless, unlovable, and wounded. Then we drive people further away, leaving ourselves more lonely and isolated than before.

The behaviors and patterns that are harmful and destructive to our relationships are also harmful to us. We harm ourselves when we settle for less than we want or deserve. And we certainly injure ourselves when we believe that we're responsible for others' abusive behavior. When we deny or minimize abuse, we give ourselves the message that we're not worth believing and not valuable enough to be treated kindly.

Women harm themselves in a variety of other ways too. Unfortunately we can be versatile in the ways we treat ourselves unkindly or unfairly. We may hate our bodies and our appearance. We may berate ourselves for not progressing faster in our recovery. We expect ourselves to be perfect and criticize ourselves mercilessly when we're not.

The next time you tell yourself you're worthless, hopeless, neurotic, or to blame, think about how another woman would feel if you made the same comments to her. You'd owe her amends for your harsh judgments. Consider treating yourself with the same consideration. Put your name on your list of Eighth Step amends and begin healing your relationship with *yourself*.

SIMPLE BUT NOT EASY

Making a list of amends may sound like a simple activity, but there's a lot involved. Besides discovering our true responsibility in each situation, it can be painful to think about our relationships. We may feel sad or disturbed recalling past events.

Constance found Step Eight difficult because she had to acknowledge things in the past she could not change. It was a time for grieving and tears. She was especially sad about the breakup of a romantic relationship that had lasted ten years. She regretted the things she had done to contribute to the breakup and wished she could go back and undo her past actions. Step Eight allowed her to experience her sadness, grieve her loss, and forgive herself in a way she hadn't before.

Mary Lynn's experience was similar. Her mother had become disabled when Mary Lynn was a child. Because her mother was unable to care for her, Mary Lynn had resented her most of her life. As she considered this relationship in Step Eight, she realized no one could ever give her the mothering she'd always wanted. Letting go of the past, she mourned the loss of the mother-daughter relationship she had so deeply desired.

If you find it difficult to explore your relationships at Step Eight, remember you can approach them one at a time. Go slowly and remember everything you've learned from previous Steps: a spiritual presence accepts you just as you are; you don't have to be perfect; you can ask for and receive compassionate help.

It's a good idea to get support from other women while doing this Step, particularly from women who've been in situations similar to yours. If it's painful to think about your relationship with your children, you might want to seek out another woman with children. If you have a history of sexual abuse, find other women who share your experience.

One caution: Make sure you find someone who acknowledges that harm is a *shared* responsibility. Some people in recovery programs might balk at the suggestion that we hold others accountable for what they've done to us. Traditionally, AA holds that we set the other person's actions aside and "sweep off our side of the street."[3]

But when we don't hold others accountable, we're often too ready to believe that we caused or provoked someone else's behavior

—or even deserved the abuse we received. Sometimes it seems easier to say, "I'm sorry," than to say, "I didn't like what you did and here's how I reacted. I hope we can work out a better relationship. Here's what I'm willing to do."

Of course, we need to assume responsibility when we *are* to blame. But it's equally important to recognize where we're *not* to blame. We can look to people who will support us unconditionally as we explore each relationship and discover this balance for ourselves.

THE ART OF WILLINGNESS

Making a list of amends is only the beginning of Step Eight. Willingness follows. Willingness involves gaining truth and clarity about our relationships. With this wisdom, we can begin to make things right, to relate in a new way.

I procrastinated taking Step Eight because I was worried about making amends. How was I going to approach the people on my list? Fortunately, my sponsor reminded me about willingness: Step Eight asks that I become willing. I don't have to worry about *making* amends—the next Step—until I'm ready.

How do we develop willingness? In much the same way we "became entirely ready" to let go of our old patterns in Step Six. Just as we looked at each pattern in Step Six and asked ourselves what prevented us from giving it up, in Step Eight we can look at each name on our list of amends and ask, What stands in my way of clearing out the negativity in this relationship?

You may find that nothing stands in your way with some of the people on your list. You may be prepared to move forward and make your amends. But when you think about becoming more open or honest with others, you may feel anxiety or dread or full-blown panic. If you react this way, be gentle with yourself. Trust that as you gain truthfulness and clarity, your inner knowing will guide you as you consider making peace with each person.

Take a step back and ask yourself some questions: Is there an old pattern that prevents me from being honest in this relationship? Am I still trying to please or control or behave in another way that interferes with an honest relationship? If so, walk through Steps Six and Seven again. Or you may want to go back to Step Four to see if you missed something in your inventory.

If you aren't willing to make amends to a particular person, let it go for a time. Move ahead with the amends you are willing to make, and be patient with yourself for the others. The time will come. You may find that when you do some of your easier Ninth Step amends you will become willing to make amends that seem impossible right now.

In Step Eight we keep an open mind. We take time to learn more about ourselves. The challenges we face in Step Eight lead us to a deeper understanding of ourselves and prepare us for a new way of relating to the world.

Step Nine

*Made direct amends to such people wherever possible,
except when to do so would injure them or others.*

STEP NINE MOVES US into the present. It asks us to take action
with what we've learned in Step Eight. Most of us look at Step Nine
and wonder how we'll ever be able to do it. We can usually think
of at least one or two people and past events—maybe several—we'd
rather forget or avoid entirely. We may feel vulnerable and afraid,
doubting that we'll be able to be honest with the people we most
need to approach.

Earlier Steps have taught us that fear doesn't have to stop us
from moving ahead. If we wait for the fear to go away, we may find
ourselves waiting a long time to make our amends. Instead, we can
use the inner and outer resources we've developed in our recovery
to help us find the courage to act in the face of fear. The other Steps
are a foundation supporting us through our Ninth Step amends.

What does it mean to make amends to another person? It
means taking responsibility for your part in a relationship.
Responsibility refers to the ability to respond appropriately. When
you do, you extend hope for something new to yourself and to
another person. You may even find that your "enemies" become
your friends.

To begin making amends, look at each name on your list and decide what you need to do to re-create the best possible relationship with that person. A direct discussion may be the best approach in some cases. In others, you may make "living amends" by practicing new behavior. Your amends may be as simple as adopting a new attitude toward someone on your list. Or it might mean not including a certain person in your life anymore. Each situation is unique; no two amends are alike.

CLEARING THE PAST

Sometimes making amends means directly apologizing or expressing regret for something we've done. We've often hurt people and damaged our relationships when we've pursued our cravings at all costs. In Step Eight we identified the people we had harmed, either by directly embarrassing, threatening, or frightening them or by indirectly trying to control them. Now we have a chance to re-create or renew our relationships.

Natalie made amends to her boyfriend for her out-of-control drinking behavior which had caused him great concern. "He was relieved to hear me take responsibility for my actions and grateful to know that he wasn't to blame," she says. "Now we both agree that I'm responsible for myself."

Many of us have financial amends to make if we've stolen money or acquired things dishonestly. Jackie, who shopped compulsively and ran up a large debt, sent anonymous payments to businesses where she'd shoplifted merchandise or used false credit to buy clothes or furniture. Other women have repaid their employers for items they've stolen. One woman repaid a large sum of money she received for a project she never completed. Step Nine gives us the opportunity to make restitution, to pay back debts like these and become financially responsible.

Some amends are symbolic. Sometimes we can't speak to or visit someone on our list. We frequently lose contact with people because they've moved away or perhaps died, making direct amends impossible. Or we may owe amends to an institution, such as a church or the courts, because we've been dishonest or disrespectful. Natalie, for instance, lied about her financial status to receive financial aid in college. How do we make amends in these situations?

If we can't go directly to the person to whom we owe amends, we can find a way to do something generous or helpful instead—give money to a charity, plant a tree, write a poem, do whatever allows us to set things right and restore balance. Natalie donated money to a scholarship fund. Constance, whose father died, wrote him a letter and read it to her sponsor.

My friend Grace values these symbolic amends. "Our desire for healing or peace in a relationship is profound, even when we can't act on it directly," she says. "I feel like I'm erasing my footsteps and restoring balance when I make symbolic amends."

"LIVING AMENDS"

Direct and honest amends usually involve a spoken apology or direct action. But sometimes indirect or "living" amends are more appropriate. Amends are about setting things right, making peace with another person. What actions can we take to restore balance to our relationships? We may simply choose to begin treating someone with more respect or kindness than we have in the past.

Eve felt she'd never be able to make amends to her ex-husband. She eventually realized that a formal meeting to discuss their relationship wasn't necessary. Instead, she made living amends to him by no longer reacting as she always had. Rather than criticizing him at every opportunity, she treats him respectfully and cooperates with their child visitation arrangement. To her amazement, he's more cooperative in return.

Similarly, Lois started having casual conversations with people at work whom she had avoided for years. It didn't seem necessary to make formal amends for her rudeness, but she wanted to be more civil toward her co-workers. Now she says hello or has a friendly chat with people she purposely avoided in the past.

Elena made living amends to her two brothers. She was with them while their mother was dying, and she consciously chose to let her brothers react in their own ways, without trying to take care of them or change them. Elena's brothers had difficulty expressing their feelings about their mother's condition. She would have preferred that they discuss openly what was happening and support each other, but Elena recognized her brothers' right to grieve in their own ways. She believed her attitude of acceptance was the most loving amends she could make.

Many women talk about making living amends with their children by becoming better parents—treating their children with more attentiveness, consistency, and maturity.

Elena, for instance, realized that she'd begun making amends with her five-year-old daughter when her daughter's teacher commented on how calm and relaxed the little girl had become. Elena had not made direct amends to her daughter, but she had begun spending more time with her and interacting with her in a healthier way. In fact, as the quality of Elena's emotional life improved, as she became less moody and anxious, so did her daughter.

While many of us tell our children we're sorry for the things we've done or not done, the words are only part of the amends. The power of making amends to a child or anyone else lies in the follow-through, the actions that back up our words. Words of apology or explanation can be meaningless, especially if the children are very young or if our actions don't reflect our words.

CONSIDERING OUR MOTIVES

Our amends are intended to clear away the "wreckage of the past."[1] Before we proceed with our amends, we need to consider carefully *why* we want to make amends to a particular person.

In Step Eight we talked about how women often feel compelled to apologize, and I encourage you to keep that in mind now too. Do you want to make amends because you owe an apology, or are you trying to control a difficult relationship by giving in or taking blame? Is your apology a way to gain acceptance or love from someone else? Are you hoping the other person will feel guilty or sympathetic or make amends to you in return?

Even if you are genuinely atoning for your behavior, take a deep look inside to see if you're hoping for a specific response from the other person. Hidden motives will affect the way you make amends and can add to the wreckage you hope to remove. For instance, you can admit to a friend that you've been sarcastic with her, but you can say this in a dozen different ways. If you're secretly hoping to vent your anger, you will communicate anger in your amends. For example, you might say, "I've noticed that I'm often sarcastic with you when you're feeling sorry for yourself." This statement may honestly describe your behavior, but it also insults your friend. It might be more constructive to say, "I know I've been sarcastic with you, usually when I've been afraid to say how I really feel. I want to be more honest. Even if I can't be, I'll try not to use sarcasm to make my point."

We want to be honest when making our amends, but we can choose *how* to be truthful. The intent of our amends is to bring our relationships back to balance—to make things right, not to further damage them. In Twelve Step meetings you'll often hear that honesty without sensitivity is brutality. Our underlying motives will influence the way we tell the truth.

It's helpful to stop and think about what we're trying to accomplish in our Ninth Step amends. Do we have a hidden motive? What do we imagine will happen? If we worry too much about the other person's response—whether he or she will be grateful or angry or tearful—we'll lose sight of the real intention of this Step: to focus on *our* responsibility in the relationship. What can *we* say or do to take responsibility for our part in the relationship?

LETTING GO OF THE OUTCOME

In the Ninth Step our only obligation is to take the action we think right and let go of the outcome. The truth is, *we have no control over the other person's response* when we make amends. We do what we can to set the relationship right and surrender the outcome.

One woman owed her ex-husband financial amends. He had overpaid for child support, and she owed him a large sum. At first she decided not to tell him about it, but her guilt increased as time went on. Finally she accepted her responsibility to reimburse him for the overpayment. When she made amends and offered to repay him, he was furious that she thought he had made a mistake. He wouldn't accept the repayment!

We can't predict how people will respond to our amends. They may accept them with love and relief, they may ignore or minimize them, or they may become self-righteous and angry because we've finally admitted what they suspected about us all along. But if we are clear, open, and honest about our responsibility in a relationship, we've done our part to set things right.

One of Ruth's first amends included a visit to the people who hosted the party where Ruth, the guest of honor, ended the evening passed out on the floor while the guests stepped over her on their way out. The hosts were delighted to hear that Ruth was finally sober. They had been concerned about her and accepted her amends with good humor and compassion. They all laughed heartily over the absurdity of Ruth's last drunk.

Elena, on the other hand, found that people aren't always receptive to amends. When she approached her younger sister to admit how she had carelessly involved her in a number of compromising sexual situations years before, her sister didn't want to talk about it. "She said it was no big deal and wouldn't sit still to listen to me," Elena recalls.

Elena is glad she opened up to her sister. "At least she knows I'm aware I hurt her," she says. "I hope the time will come when we'll be able to talk together. Sometimes it's hard to accept that the past isn't resolved at the pace I'd like."

We can do only our part when making amends. At times our best intentions will get little or no response. Still, we make the effort. We offer honesty and clarity and release control over the outcome.

INJURING OTHERS

The Ninth Step says we refrain from making amends to others "when to do so would injure them or others." How can amends cause injury? When the authors of the Twelve Steps wrote Step Nine, they were concerned that in our efforts to be "rigorously honest," we might disclose incidents or indiscretions better left unmentioned.

If you've had an affair with a married man and his wife doesn't know about it, you'll only injure the wife by going to her to confess your behavior. If you've been saying cruel things about a co-worker to your boss, your co-worker would probably be injured if you revealed your thoughtlessness. It may be better to go to your boss with your amends rather than to apologize to your co-worker. This is the spirit of avoiding injury to others.

Those of us with children need to be cautious about injuring our children with our amends. We might want to admit everything we think we've done wrong as their mother. But before we do, we need to ask ourselves who will benefit. We might feel some relief from that gnawing "mother guilt," but we may risk overwhelming our children with information. They will benefit more if we make general amends and *act* on our words by becoming more loving, caring, and considerate parents.

There is a time to let go of the guilt. Each of us will discover the right time for ourselves. One woman shared in an Al-Anon meeting that her mother, a recovering alcoholic, was still making amends to her for things that had happened many years before. The daughter was ready to forgive and move on, but her mother felt guilty and could not let go and accept that she could not change her past behavior. The mother's never-ending amends *interfered* with their relationship. The daughter was burdened with her mother's regret and remorse and wondered how she could convince her mother that she forgave her.

With my own children, I try to sense when I am apologizing too much. I am learning to respect their limits, knowing that I risk putting them in the awkward position of taking care of me when I am feeling guilty.

We sometimes find that people react strongly when we make amends. When this happens, we want to be careful about how we interpret "injury." Hurt feelings and strong reactions don't necessarily mean we've injured someone. This is especially important for women to remember; we are often too worried about pleasing other people. It's possible to become too focused on the chances of injuring people and to forget that "negative" emotions might be a normal response to our amends. In fact, we might find greater healing and openness when we work through the anger and sorrow that arise.

RESPECTING FEELINGS—
INCLUDING OUR OWN

Sometimes our amends stir up unpleasant memories of the past. If this happens, we must be gentle and wait. Perhaps others are not yet ready to hear what we have to say.

Mary Lynn wanted to make amends with her parents. When she was addicted to alcohol and drugs in her adolescence, she went through a frightening period of self-destructive behavior. Her parents placed her in institutional care at age sixteen. Mary Lynn found it was too painful for her family to talk about this traumatic time. She waited for ten years until her family was finally able to discuss those painful events and accept her amends.

When they were ready, Mary Lynn's father told her he'd felt helpless and afraid as he watched Mary Lynn nearly kill herself with alcohol and narcotics. She saw a vulnerable and compassionate side of her father she'd never seen before. Mary Lynn had been uncomfortable waiting so long to make this amends, but she now understood her parents' unwillingness to discuss the past. The experience renewed her respect and love for them, and a more honest relationship began to develop.

Sometimes our amends redefine the past. When our amends include being honest about our feelings, we may need to strike a delicate balance between others' feelings and our own. For instance, if we've spent years being emotionally dishonest—hiding our feelings—we may make amends by speaking up for ourselves or asking for what we need. People around us might not welcome the change.

Making amends with our families might involve saying no when we don't want to run an errand, fix a meal, or do a load of laundry when someone asks us to. If we've always said yes to please others, our family members might react with anger or displeasure when we set limits.

Our partner or children may feel inconvenienced and bothered by our behavior, but their protests don't mean we're causing injury—or that their feelings are more important than ours. We can respect our own feelings. If we try to make peace by continuing to pretend we're satisfied with our role, we risk continuing the emotional dishonesty that led to our amends in the first place.

Becoming honest and setting boundaries often involves working through some conflict. Some resistance to change is natural when we start to redefine our role in a relationship. We can respectfully acknowledge the fears of those around us as we renew and re-create our relationships in the present by making amends.

MAKING AMENDS TO OURSELVES

Including ourselves on our Eighth Step list of amends gives us the opportunity to begin making amends to ourselves. In fact, our recovery is the living amends we make to ourselves. Becoming sober and abstinent, working the Steps, and giving ourselves a chance to live differently begin healing the harm done to our self-esteem, our bodies, and our relationships.

Participating in our recovery is only one way we make living amends to ourselves. If we are habitually self-critical, we may want to affirm ourselves with positive messages. Or we may simply practice self-acceptance by *observing* our actions rather than *judging* them. For instance, I can observe, "I'm starting to act helpless and shy to get attention" rather than judging myself, "There I go again! Am I ever going to act like a normal human being?" When we remember that we don't have to be perfect and that we have permission to make mistakes, we make amends to ourselves.

Many of us have harmed our bodies with years of compulsive dieting, chronic stress, or too much drinking or drug use. It's likely our bodies have taken abuse and need special attention to return to health and strength. We can make amends by treating our bodies with new respect—eating well, exercising, and getting enough rest.

Many of us feel ashamed of our bodies. Then we numb our shame with our drug of choice, or we starve, purge, or take diet pills to "fix" our bodies. Either way, we hurt ourselves trying to achieve the ideal body, and we feel depressed and anxious when our bodies are less than "perfect." Amends to ourselves might include accepting our bodies as they are, rather than automatically assuming our bodies are inadequate or flawed.

For some of us, making amends to ourselves means having more discipline—paying bills on time or keeping commitments. When we act responsibly, our lives become easier. For others, it may mean relaxing a bit, allowing ourselves the luxury of letting some projects go unfinished. If we're overachievers, we may feel much better about ourselves if we allow ourselves to do less. That was my own lesson in making amends to myself: I could take better care of myself by letting go of my need to do the most and the best of everything.

A manageable life, care for our bodies, and participating in our recovery are amends we owe ourselves.

A NEW FREEDOM AND A NEW HAPPINESS

When we begin to make amends, we may feel overwhelmed. Step Nine does take courage and effort. But according to the AA Big Book, "we are going to know a new freedom and a new happiness."[2]

Our fear of the past will diminish because we've taken a clear and honest look at our lives. People can now come closer; we don't have to run or hide. We make amends so that we can begin to have relationships full of life and truth and trust. Poet Adrienne Rich describes the possibilities inherent in this kind of relationship:

> *It isn't that to have an honorable relationship with you, I have to understand everything, or tell you everything at once, or that I can know, beforehand, everything I need to tell you.*
>
> *It means that most of the time I am eager, longing for the possibility of telling you. That these possibilities may seem frightening, but not destructive, to me. That I feel strong enough to hear your tentative and groping words. That we both*

know we are trying, all the time, to extend the possibilities of truth between us.

The possibility of life between us.[3]

Once we begin making amends, we'll realize how much remorse, guilt, and resentment we've been carrying. Having turned the light on these obstacles, we no longer stumble over the "wreckage of the past."

Making amends, we'll experience another paradox of recovery: strength and serenity come from humility and vulnerability. We gain strength when we let other people see us as we are. We gain honor and respect for ourselves when we are open and honest and responsible, able to respond appropriately.

As we dare to tell the truth, we start to participate more fully in life. We create a healthy environment in which our old patterns are less likely to reemerge. When we heal the past—setting our relationships right—we take the Ninth Step out of the old life and into the new.

Step Ten

*Continued to take personal inventory
and when we were wrong promptly admitted it.*

STEP TEN IS THE FIRST OF THE THREE MAINTENANCE STEPS. By practicing a regular inventory in Step Ten, we keep ourselves aware and focused in the present.

We've done lots of challenging work as we've gone through the Steps so far. As much as we might want to slow down, relax, or even stop, we need to be careful about sliding back into old habits and patterns. That's why we practice a regular check-in in Step Ten; the observation and self-reflection monitor our lives and relationships in the present. This Step keeps us focused on living each moment in a spiritual way and maintaining the progress we've already made.

If we think of Steps One through Nine as being similar to a physical checkup, Step Ten would be the routine we create afterward to keep our bodies in good health. When we get a checkup we discover where our bodies need special attention. Then we begin the daily practices that will bring us optimum health. If we exercise, eat right, and minimize stress, our physical condition will be healthier.

In Step Ten we begin the daily practices that will bring us the greatest *emotional* and *spiritual* health. We gained awareness from previous Steps about where to place our attention. Now we make a daily commitment to continuing observation and reflection—recognizing when we're out of balance or hurting ourselves or others. Our ongoing awareness allows us to meet each day and each relationship with responsibility. Without daily reflection, we risk the emotional turmoil—new resentments, worries, jealousies, and fears—that can push us back into our old behaviors.

AA says that we have a "daily reprieve" from our drinking as long as we continue to practice what we've learned so far in recovery. We've taken the Steps to understand the past and take responsibility for ourselves. Now we apply what we've learned to the present.

GETTING CURRENT

In Step Ten we practice taking inventory of the things that are happening in our lives today, giving up our unwanted patterns and making amends right away. Some of us find it helpful to share our insights with someone else, as we did in Step Five.

Many women do a formal Tenth Step every day, others once a week or at some other regular interval. Some of us take a more informal approach, continually reflecting on our lives with an intuition or inner knowing that tells us when to stop and pay closer attention to a particular situation.

Sex and Love Addicts Anonymous calls this regular inventory process "getting current." Whether we do it every night or whenever it's needed, the Tenth Step inventory helps us look at what's going on in our lives in the moment. Where are we in danger of slipping back into a destructive pattern or perhaps creating a new one? Where are we being dishonest with ourselves or someone else? How are we feeling about ourselves today? Is there anything that doesn't feel finished?

By doing a Tenth Step, we avoid creating new wreckage with unfinished business that ends up blocking our path today. Step Ten gives us an opportunity to set things right in our relationships as we go along, rather than piling up resentments and regrets.

One evening Francesca was busy waiting on a customer during the dinnertime rush and responded sharply when another waiter asked her a question. Reflecting later, Francesca regretted her response, realizing that it would have been simple enough to have said she was too busy to talk. The next day, she apologized to her co-worker for her curtness.

"I don't know if she accepted my apology or not, but I felt better acknowledging that I could have acted differently," says Francesca. "When I make a Tenth Step amends like this, it means that I don't have to carry around a load of guilt or remorse. I can set things right and let it go. Even the smallest amends make a big difference."

PUTTING THE DAY TO BED

Like many women, Norma practices a nightly Tenth Step and thoughtfully reviews her day. She calls it "putting the day to bed." This self-reflection may come easily, because many of us are naturally introspective and spontaneously reflect on what's happening in our lives and what it means. We can think of a Tenth Step as an extension of the reflective activities we may already do: keeping a journal, talking through an issue with a therapist, turning to a friend to help us sort out our feelings.

At first Norma wrote in her journal each night, describing the confusing or troubling things that had happened during the day. Then she would reflect on each instance, asking herself if she was doing everything she could to be honest and responsible.

Remember that *responsibility* means "the ability to respond." When we're responsible we don't necessarily fix or take care of things, we respond appropriately. For Norma this means taking action in some situations and doing nothing in others. For instance, she refused to loan a sum of money to her niece. When her niece became resentful and angry, Norma wondered if she had been responsible. She was tempted to make amends.

In reflecting on her decision in her nightly Tenth Step, Norma concluded she had acted appropriately by refusing her niece in a gentle way. Her reflection allowed her to live with the tension in the relationship and to let her niece have her feelings. We sometimes find as we review a situation with our Tenth Step that there's nothing to do but let it be or let it go.

After this nightly Tenth Step became routine, Norma found herself spontaneously reviewing her day without needing to write everything down. Now she sees the Tenth Step as *a way of thinking* rather than a formal exercise. She's established a practice that helps her stay balanced and aware in her recovery.

LIKE THE LAYERS OF AN ONION

The Tenth Step leads us to understand and accept ourselves at deeper and deeper levels. We'll hear recovering women talk about this discovery process as peeling away the layers of an onion. Under one layer is another and then another. "More will be revealed" is a popular AA saying.

As you review each day, you may see patterns you didn't know existed, or you may discover new features in the patterns you've already identified. Maybe you'll realize for the first time that authority figures tend to trigger your rebellious behavior. Or maybe you'll notice that your urge to take charge of other people's lives is strongest when you're around your parents; perhaps you'll recognize a need to show them how competent you are or to protect yourself from their controlling tendencies.

When we review our reactions that arise each day—in conversations and interactions with other people—we receive plenty of information about how we respond to life. Everyday events can be like mirrors that reflect our deeper selves. With them, we can more thoroughly understand our deepest values and feelings. If we practice this Step in a spirit of gentle observation and self-acceptance, we'll release more guilt, confusion, and shame.

In the Tenth Step we "continue to watch for selfishness, dishonesty, resentment, and fear," the Big Book tells us. "When these crop up, we ask God at once to remove them."[1] Women often find that these "defects" become more manageable as we work with these feelings and behaviors and reflect on them more deeply.

I found out for myself that a Tenth Step can help me discover *the feeling underneath the feeling.* A few years into my recovery, I became involved in a relationship where I felt chronically angry and unhappy. In my daily Tenth Step I easily identified the anger and assumed I shouldn't be experiencing it. After all, the AA Big Book tells me that anger is the "dubious luxury of normal men"[2] and can lead an alcoholic straight back to drinking. I struggled to release the anger but found it persisted. Then I stopped to ask myself what it might be covering up.

I found I felt terribly hurt under my anger. The angry feelings protected me from the pain underneath. When I stopped focusing on removing the anger and asked myself what the anger was about, I started being truthful with myself and my partner about why I was feeling hurt. Then anger was no longer an issue.

Truth is the theme of the Tenth Step. To keep this in mind, we can think about this Step as Jackie does: "I continue to take a personal inventory of my truth and promptly admit it, no matter what I find." Jackie's interpretation of this Step urges us to peel away more layers. "Go deeper with the truth and always honor it, even if it feels uncomfortable or difficult," she says.

The Tenth Step is particularly powerful for women. We have a chance to unconditionally accept and validate *our experience*. As women, we often find that few people stop to ask us how we're feeling or how we're responding to the day's events, but we can give this gift to ourselves. As we review each day we can ask, What did I notice today? What did I recognize about myself and others? What was true for *me* today? What do I believe?

This can be especially important if we come from families that denied our experience. Those of us from abusive homes, for example, may find our families try to pretend that there was no abuse and often punish or reject family members who disagree. As a result, recognizing abuse—even admitting it to ourselves—can often be too frightening and threatening. We may start to believe the family lies about abuse and doubt our own feelings and perceptions. When we have this kind of history, the Tenth Step can help us regain trust in our own experience.

No matter what our background, the Tenth Step can help us affirm ourselves and our experience. Admitting the truth to ourselves empowers us to live a spiritual life—to be fully who we are.

WHEN ARE WE WRONG?

Step Ten says we promptly acknowledge "when we were wrong." Why is this important? As in Step Five, admitting our wrongs allows us to connect humbly with another human being. We extend the risk we took when we admitted our wrongs to one trusted person to other relationships in our lives. This new way of living invites others to be less afraid, and more open and honest in return.

Vivian learned the value of admitting wrong after she'd received a traffic ticket when she failed to stop for a pedestrian in a crosswalk. For a while Vivian blamed everyone else for the incident. Finally she admitted it had been her fault. It was a humbling experience, but admitting her mistake gave her a new kind of freedom. She realized she could admit her wrong and not feel obliged to hide in shame.

"I accepted it as a human error that anyone could have made," she says. "It didn't mean that I was bad or inadequate or unfit to participate in society. This was a new concept for me. I had thought that making mistakes meant *I was* a mistake. So I always had to be perfect—and *right*. I could admit my fault and still accept myself. This showed me how far I'd come in my recovery."

As we've seen in several other Steps, we want to be very careful about how we apply the word *wrong* to ourselves. We don't want to generalize and always assume we're wrong just because someone else says we are. It's important to reflect on each situation and determine our true accountability. We have to be careful not to assume we're wrong when we feel hurt or angry about someone else's behavior.

The traditional AA view is that when "somebody hurts us and we feel sore, we are in the wrong also."[3] It's important that women look a little deeper so that we don't interpret this in a self-blaming way. Too many of us will readily assume we're wrong whenever a conflict arises or someone attacks or offends us. For women, it is important to practice *not* making ourselves wrong and to concentrate instead on how we feel.

Feeling hurt or angry about someone else's actions has nothing to do with right or wrong. If we're upset with someone, our emotional reactions are acceptable and valid, no matter what they are. If we choose to act on our feelings in a vengeful or manipulative way, we miss the point of Step Ten, and we may have some regrets later on. But the feelings themselves are not wrong. We can let ourselves feel what we feel. And we can ask ourselves why we're having such an intense emotional response and what this person's behavior means to us. This is our truth.

Still, if we become consumed with anger or resentment, we throw ourselves off balance and make things worse for ourselves. To maintain our sanity and sobriety we often need to find constructive ways to express or release our feelings and take care of ourselves. And we can remember to go deeper with a feeling before we try to make it go away.

WHAT WE "OWN" AND WHAT WE DON'T

A Tenth Step is a review of the day or week or moment, or whatever time interval we choose, that helps us reflect on what we "own" and what we don't. Just as in Step Nine, we can determine our responsibility, do what is necessary to set things right, and let go of the outcome. In many cases there may be nothing to do, or it may be that someone else "owns" the problem.

A painful or uncomfortable situation may remain painful because you don't "own" the problem and can't do anything to fix it. Sometimes natural tension results when two people disagree. Perhaps you and your lover have discovered that your values on a sensitive issue differ. Maybe your children are furious because you've set limits they don't like.

When we become truthful with ourselves in our Tenth Step, we become more truthful with others. This sometimes creates disagreements we might prefer to avoid. Admitting we were wrong may heighten the discomfort or conflict in a relationship because honesty brings the conflict out into the open.

As we reflect with a Tenth Step on situations like these, we may find it appropriate simply to accept the conflict that inevitably arises in relationships. As difficult as this may be, we must sometimes let go of the outcome and let other people—and ourselves—feel unhappy, angry, or disappointed.

When doing her Tenth Step, Constance asks herself how she has been indirect today. She acknowledges her habit of not speaking up for herself. In her eagerness to please other people, she frequently tries to tolerate conditions that are unacceptable to her. When she recognizes that she has been too accommodating, she asks herself if admitting her wrong means speaking with the other person.

One evening Constance went to meet her friend Cindy for dinner, but Cindy never showed up. Constance was hurt, but she instinctively blamed herself for her friend's thoughtlessness. "I must not be good company; otherwise Cindy would have remembered our date," she thought.

At first, Constance decided to say nothing, but when she did her Tenth Step inventory she realized she was being disrespectful to herself. She was letting herself be treated carelessly. When she finally confronted Cindy with her disappointment and hurt, Cindy told her she was too sensitive and overreacting. As a result, their friendship cooled. But Constance felt she owed it to herself to be honest about her feelings. The alternative—convincing herself her feelings were wrong or unimportant—was more hurtful.

WALKING DOWN ANOTHER STREET

One of the best things about Step Ten is that you already know how to do it. There's nothing in Step Ten you haven't done in the other Steps. In this Step you refine what you've learned so far and practice applying it to your daily life.

If you begin your Tenth Step practice by writing each night or creating another regular routine, you'll probably find that the self-reflection inventory process becomes second nature after a while. You'll develop a natural ability to sense when you're losing your emotional balance or harming yourself or someone else. Then you can pause, reflect, and ask yourself, What is my appropriate response? What can I do to set things right?

When you practice the Tenth Step you find yourself living in the present moment and becoming more self-aware and spontaneous. What a contrast to the days when we were habitually frightened, controlling, and numb!

The Tenth Step is at the heart of our personal power—changing what we can, accepting what we can't change, and developing a growing wisdom to know the difference. Now we can participate in life and trust that we'll have options and choices when problems or conflicts arise. Now we can be responsible—able to respond—because we no longer cling to our old patterns. We may still fall back into them once in awhile, but we know how to climb back out, as Portia Nelson acknowledges in her poem "Autobiography in Five Short Chapters":

I

I walk down the street.
> There is a deep hole in the sidewalk.
> I fall in.
> I am lost…I am helpless.
>> It isn't my fault.
> It takes forever to find a way out.

II

I walk down the same street.

There is a deep hole in the sidewalk.

I pretend I don't see it.

I fall in again.

I can't believe I am in this same place.

But, it isn't my fault.

It still takes a long time to get out.

III

I walk down the same street.

There is a deep hole in the sidewalk.

I *see* it there.

I still fall in…it's a habit…but,

my eyes are open.

I know where I am.

It is *my* fault.

I get out immediately.

IV

I walk down the same street.

There is a deep hole in the sidewalk.

I walk around it.

V

I walk down another street.[4]

Step Eleven

Sought through prayer and meditation to improve our conscious contact with God as we understood Him, praying only for knowledge of His will for us and the power to carry that out.

STEP ELEVEN ENCOURAGES US TO TURN INWARD and deepen our awareness of our Higher Power by setting aside time for prayer and meditation. These practices lead us to reach for whatever we believe is greater than, deeper than, or beyond ourselves. Prayer and meditation can bring us serenity—moments, hours, maybe even days of it—that we perhaps have never experienced before. We can also practice prayer and meditation to regain our emotional balance when confronted with events or relationships that worry or upset us.

The Eleventh Step can show you how far you've come along the path of spiritual growth. If you were angry at religion or doubtful about a spiritual essence—a Goddess, Higher Power, Higher Self, or Life Force—that supports you, ask yourself how you're feeling now. Do you sense a new awareness of your connection with other people and with the greater web of life itself?

We need to give our attention to this spiritual connection day by day so it will thrive and flourish. It's like starting a garden and then tending it properly so it will grow and be fruitful. We wouldn't set out seedlings and then neglect them, hoping for enough rainfall to keep them alive. Instead, we need to watch them every day, water them regularly, and give them extra nutrients and protection when they need it.

Similarly, we can't take our spiritual life for granted or assume it will take care of itself without any special effort on our part. To stay healthy and strong, our spiritual connection needs our ongoing attention. This means consciously taking time to nurture the central relationship of our lives: the relationship between ourselves and our healing or guiding spirit. We began developing this relationship in Step Three; now we cultivate it with time and attention in Step Eleven.

This is what "improving our conscious contact" means. We cultivate conscious contact with a power greater than ourselves through practices such as prayer and meditation.

PERSONALIZING OUR PRAYERS

Prayer is an act of either reaching out to a Higher Power or going inward to a deeper knowing. Just as we described God in our own way in Step Three, we can also come to prayer however we like. Our willingness to pray and be open to this connection is more important than how we do it. *It is the spirit of our action that counts.* We can create personal rituals that symbolically open a dialogue between ourselves and the Power or Presence that supports and sustains us.

Grace believes that prayer lets her reach out to and create a relationship with her Higher Power. "In prayer I am entering into a conversation," she says. "I'm asking aloud, What do I need from the universe and what does it need from me?"

Like Grace, we can think of prayer as offering words or thoughts to our Higher Power and requesting guidance. We can create our own prayers, or we can use one of several AA prayers. As we discussed in Step Seven, if we're uncomfortable with the language of AA's prayers, we can use our own language to say precisely what we want to say.

Jackie has reworked one of AA's standard prayers—the Third Step Prayer—to include words that are meaningful and affirming for her. Although she says she started out feeling like a heretic revising this prayer, she finds that she has created a powerful sense of safety and support for herself by having the courage to personalize it.

In its original wording the Third Step prayer reads

> *God, I offer myself to Thee—to build with me and do with me as Thou wilt. Relieve me of the bondage of self, that I may better do Thy will. Take away my difficulties, that victory over them may bear witness to those I would help of Thy Power, Thy Love, and Thy Way of life. May I do Thy will always.*[1]

Jackie objects to phrases like "do with me as Thou wilt" because they remind her of her negative experiences in past relationships. She uses the word "Goddess" so that her prayer acknowledges the feminine aspect of spirituality that is important to her. Just by changing a few words, she makes this prayer more accessible and relevant for her.

Jackie's version says

Goddess, I open myself to you to work in my life today, according to divine will. Remove me from the bondage of fear, shame, and low self-esteem that I might become a channel for joy, love, and peace in the universe. Remove my difficulties as you see fit, so that victory over them would bear witness to those I would help of your love and power.

You might also find either the Seventh or the Eleventh Step Prayer from AA helpful as a basis for creating a prayer that honors your individual experience.

The traditional Seventh Step Prayer (see page 113) focuses on character defects, so it might be appropriate if you want to concentrate on giving up behaviors or attitudes that trouble you. You might want to choose another word for "defects," one with a more positive or neutral meaning, such as "patterns."

The Eleventh Step Prayer is an adaptation of a prayer written by St. Francis of Assisi. It beautifully expresses a desire to create a positive environment in our lives. We want to be cautious, however, about following its suggestion about "self-forgetting," so we don't minimize the importance of seeking help for ourselves.

Lord, make me a channel of thy peace—that where there is hatred, I may bring love—that where there is wrong, I may bring the spirit of forgiveness—that where there is discord, I may bring harmony—that where there is error, I may bring truth—that where there is doubt, I may bring faith—that where there is despair, I may bring hope—that where there are shadows, I may bring light—that where there is sadness,

I may bring joy. Lord, grant that I may seek rather to comfort
than to be comforted—to love, than to be loved. For it is by
self-forgetting that one finds. It is by forgiving that one is for-
given. It is by dying that one awakens to Eternal Life.[2]

You may also find the Serenity Prayer (see page 114) is all you
need. I use this prayer on a regular basis as an Eleventh Step when
my life gets out of balance.

Of course, your prayers, if you choose to pray, may not resem-
ble these prayers at all. You may include prayers from your own
religious tradition or prayers that are composed entirely in your
own words. You may, in the tradition of Eastern religions, simply
ask for the greatest good and the spiritual best for all.

Even though Frances doesn't like to pray to ask for things, she
still prays to express her desire for the best possible outcomes in her
life. "Having a passion for what is good is still part of my spiritual
life," she says. "So prayer includes praying for my own well-being
and the well-being of others."

But beyond seeking the good, Frances thinks of prayer as "gaining awareness." To her it's a process of connecting with an accessible and available inner wisdom. By praying—saying certain words
that have special meaning for her—she reminds herself to open to
that wisdom and listen to what it has to say.

THE WILL OF THE UNIVERSE

Step Eleven says that we pray "only for knowledge of His will for
us and the power to carry that out." Ruth interprets this to mean

that there's a spirit moving the universe, and she prays to think and act in harmony with that spirit.

When Ruth reads Step Eleven, she assumes that "His will" is *the will of the universe that things be the way they are*. When we are "doing God's will," we are accepting and aware and able to act appropriately. We let go of our desire to control things we can't change.

This doesn't mean that we give in or give up when challenges arise. On the contrary, acting appropriately may involve standing up for ourselves, resisting pressure to conform to others' wishes, or witnessing for a cause we believe in. Acceptance may sometimes mean allowing other people to be angry or displeased when we set limits or start to take care of ourselves or go against the status quo.

The underlying idea is that we maintain a spirit of cooperation, letting ourselves be open to possibilities and giving up our need to know all the answers in advance.

Darlene believes the will of the universe is that she be "who I am and all that I am—and not somebody different." By practicing Step Eleven, she reminds herself she's okay just the way she is. She prays to remain open to the unknown and unseen in her life, to be responsive to whatever unfolds each day. She trusts she'll know what to do, and if she doesn't, if she makes a mistake, she'll learn something valuable.

"I believe that I'm a spiritual being and that I'm connected in ways I don't always understand," Darlene says. "I've stopped trying to figure things out in advance because I no longer see that as my job. Instead, I try to respond in the way that feels right to whatever comes to me. By giving up control like this, I've opened myself to miracles. I could never have predicted some of the best things that have happened to me in recovery."

How will we know when we're doing "God's will?" What does it feel like to cooperate with the greater forces of life? I sometimes have a feeling of "rightness"—a calm inner knowing—that tells me I'm aligned with my Higher Power. When this happens, conflicts seem to resolve themselves and I have a sense of clarity and purpose. I think of it as a state of grace.

Similarly, Maureen believes this will includes discovering what feels right and good to her, following her instincts and going where she's naturally inclined to go. This might mean doing something she enjoys—sometimes the opposite of what she thinks she's "supposed" to do. "I don't believe recovery always has to be hard," Maureen asserts. "It can seem like we're constantly required to do things that aren't fun or enjoyable in order to be doing recovery right. But I disagree. I think it's also about finding out what I love to do."

Maureen believes she is *always* doing the right thing and thinking the right thoughts. "I'm always doing God's will, no matter what I'm doing," she says. Her attitude is a variation on the recovery adage "You're exactly where you're supposed to be."

If Maureen feels anxious or worried about something, she assumes this is the way she's supposed to feel—that she's experiencing a challenge so she can learn something. If she feels overwhelmed by emotions, she looks deeper into herself to discover their source. With this attitude of self-acceptance, she avoids punishing herself for not being perfect. In her Eleventh Step, she prays to become more fully herself, to get a better and clearer sense of her place in the universe.

THE CALM IN THE CENTER

If prayer is an act of communicating, meditation is the practice of being still and *listening*. It is a time to surrender and to receive, a time to let go.

Whether you pray or not, allow yourself some meditative time each day, if only to create a peaceful moment for yourself on a regular basis.

We get very little support for quiet time in our lives. Many of us are burdened with obligations that leave us running from one responsibility to another with no time for ourselves. Others feel aimless and isolated, immobilized by depression or anxiety. Either way, we may find it difficult to direct our attention inward to listen to our inner selves.

But inner awareness is essential to our continuing growth and well-being. Because we never "graduate" from recovery, we will always be getting to know ourselves at deeper levels and adjusting to new situations and life challenges. Inner awareness evolves over time and requires our consistent attention.

If we've worked the earlier Steps and assume we've "recovered," we might forget that events will continually tempt us back into our old, destructive patterns. To protect ourselves from being drawn too far into the inevitable dramas of everyday life—where we risk becoming unbalanced again—it's important to create a "center" to return to, a serene, internal, and private place.

I have a definition of serenity that reminds me of the importance of this practice: Serenity is not freedom from the storms of life. It is the calm in the center that gets me through. We create this calm center with meditation.

Meditation is like stilling the ripples on a pond. It's quieting the mind so we can experience clarity and peace. Our daily activities and the pressures of life constantly stir up the pond, making the water turbulent and muddy. But we can calm the waters by calming ourselves, taking the time to remove ourselves from life's demands—even if just for a few minutes each day—and sit alone in stillness. In meditation we can hear ourselves *not* think.

We improve our "conscious contact" with our Higher Power or guiding spirit in stillness, by temporarily setting aside our desire to figure everything out. We acknowledge our limits and lack of control. When we sit still, we let things be. We surrender and receive.

DOING NOTHING

When we meditate, how much time is required? And what do we do when we're sitting alone and quiet? There's no one way to meditate. In fact, there are dozens of books describing different Eleventh Step meditation techniques. Just as we described God and prayer however is best for us, our meditation practice will be completely individual; we can choose from a variety of disciplines.

There are many meditation techniques that can help you set aside the nonstop chatter in your mind and quiet your thinking. You may want to sit in a chair and focus on each breath, concentrating on each inhalation and exhalation. Or you can look at a picture that calms you or gaze at a candle flame. You might repeat a mantra or affirmation, concentrating on the sound of the words to the exclusion of everything else. You might visualize a healing light, a pleasant scene, your ideal self, or an empty, quiet, peaceful space.

Sit for as long as you feel comfortable, starting with three to five minutes if that's all the time you can manage. Do whatever quiets your mind and opens a channel so you can listen to your inner self.

When we "listen" in meditation, we don't necessarily hear anything. But the act of listening itself is very important because it's a way to practice openness and receptivity. In meditation we can learn about being still, waiting to see what life brings us, and receiving it with an open heart and mind.

Ruth describes her meditation as paying attention to her breath and looking for the quiet space inside her. This helps her let go of her desire to control. "I clear away my insistence that I want or I need something and let things be," she says. "It's a new experience for me." In meditation she is willing to be present and open.

Meditation may cause some anxiety at first. When was the last time you did nothing without feeling guilty? You may find it hard to sit still. Thoughts may race through your mind as you wonder how much longer you're supposed to be meditating.

When I find myself in this state of agitation, I simply *observe* myself having these thoughts and feelings. I notice that I'm anxious. I'm aware that I'm unfocused and distressed. But I don't try to change it. I simply sit still, knowing it will pass. If the anxiety returns, I observe it again. This is a deeper level of acceptance, acceptance of *what is.*

Many women also find it helpful to make a meditative practice of walking, gardening, sewing, or painting. By doing these activities with full, conscious attention, we give ourselves a break from our usual stresses and do something good for ourselves. We can choose whatever practice gives us a sense of inner peace. And we can try to find a way to do absolutely nothing at least once in a while.

AN UNSHAKABLE FOUNDATION

In practice, prayer and meditation may not be two separate activities. We may pray while we meditate and vice versa. There's no need to distinguish the two unless it makes the practice easier. Often women talk about doing both at once.

A woman once introduced me at a conference and later confided that she had been nervous before making the introduction. To calm herself, she said, she found just a few moments to be alone. She prayed for guidance and support, seeking her inner center. This is how she regularly practices her Eleventh Step.

"Whenever I'm faced with a challenge," she told me, "I sit quietly and meditate, asking for help to get out of my own way. I ask for the strength to do what I'm here to do." By asking for guidance and sitting in silence, her meditation and prayer are completely intertwined. One flows into the other and creates a single spiritual experience.

As we start to live more consciously, we may find that prayer and meditation are spontaneous acts—we do them in the moment, as soon as we're aware we're out of balance. We begin to seek our center instinctively whenever we need it, turning toward that inner calm we've cultivated in our spiritual practices.

"There is a direct linkage among self-examination, meditation, and prayer," says AA's *Twelve Steps and Twelve Traditions*. "Taken separately, these practices can bring much relief and benefit. But when they are logically related and interwoven, the result in an unshakable foundation for life."[3]

Step Twelve

Having had a spiritual awakening as the result of these steps, we tried to carry this message to alcoholics, and to practice these principles in all our affairs.

Recovery is a new way of life. By doing our personal work in Steps One through Eleven, we develop a new way of thinking, feeling, and acting. The Twelfth Step calls this "a spiritual awakening"—awakening to a life connected to our Inner or Higher Power. It is an awakening to something greater and deeper than our own strengths and resources. That power integrates us and gives us a sense of wholeness.

During our drinking and using years, most of us felt as if we were broken into pieces that didn't quite fit together. Our addictive behavior can cause us to feel "split"—as if our feelings or actions don't belong to us. We may have been puzzled by the intensity of our own rages or depressions, or wondered why we did things that caused us shame and humiliation. It's hard to feel whole when our lives are so out of control.

BECOMING WHOLE

Becoming whole is like climbing a spiral staircase: it takes us upward but also in a circle. We're likely to pass by many of the same challenges on our way up, but they'll look different each time because we've climbed to a new level. We may find life offering opportunities to repeatedly experience old patterns and habits, but each time with more understanding. The next time the situation or pattern repeats, it will probably make more sense and be less immobilizing.

Elena now considers all of her strengths and limitations to be part of the larger fabric of her life—a tightly woven whole. "The longer I'm clean, the more comfortable I am integrating into my life the fact that I'm a drug addict," says Elena. "I'm a mother, a wife, a homemaker, a daughter, a neighbor—and a recovering cocaine user. Somehow I couldn't make all those pieces fit together before. Now it doesn't feel as if I'm leading many lives, hiding one from the other."

With the help of the Twelve Steps, we've been learning to accept and integrate the many parts of ourselves—to "own" the secrets we used to hide and to bring out our hidden strengths. By the time we reach Step Twelve, we start to feel like an integrated, complete human being. We may begin to feel balanced and centered for the first time.

This is probably not a constant feeling, just as serenity isn't a constant state we achieve. Instead, we typically experience wholeness for a moment, an hour, a day or more, then get pulled away by life's demands. But when life challenges us in this way, we can learn more about ourselves and become more deeply integrated as a result.

A SPIRITUAL AWAKENING

How do we know when we've had a spiritual awakening? What does it feel like? When does it come? Like all things spiritual, the answers will be individual. A spiritual awakening may be dramatic—a sudden experience of enlightenment—or it may be gradual and hard to describe. We might simply have a growing awareness of our connection with life and the greater whole.

We wake up spiritually in every way imaginable. When you hear stories of other women's spiritual awakenings, you can confirm and recognize your own spiritual path.

CHANGING THE PAST

Shannon's spiritual awakening came when she completed her Fourth and Fifth Steps and she realized she had changed her past. She hadn't changed any of the facts; what had happened had happened. But with a new attitude about what she'd done and what others had done to her, she forever changed her interpretation of past events. The past no longer had the power to affect her as it did before.

In letting go, Shannon felt peaceful, clear, open, and connected. She felt the shame and fear lift and sensed she was stepping into a new life. It wasn't a flash of enlightenment, but she received a sense of clarity and rightness she'd never had before.

FINDING A CALM CENTER

When Toshi went to live in Germany for a year, she felt adventurous and brave. She had been sober three years and believed she was stable enough to handle such a dramatic change. But Toshi's optimism faded soon after she arrived. She lived with a family that spoke only German, and she wasn't meeting other people easily. She felt lonely and isolated. Her adventure didn't seem like a good idea anymore. She became depressed and unsure of herself.

One day, as she was walking for hours alone and debating whether she should return home, she became aware of a tiny "speck of peace" inside her. Despite all her outer turmoil, there was a calm center. This intrigued her, and she decided to turn within rather than focus on her problems. Hers was a meditative "turning inward" experience, as we do in Step Eleven.

Toshi soon realized that this "speck" was with her wherever she went. She could turn within and find it at any time. Sometimes the speck felt expansive, and she found herself filled with an inner peace. And when it was small, it was still big enough to give her some serenity and faith, even in her most difficult moments. Finding this peaceful center was the beginning of her spiritual awakening.

CONNECTION AND ACCEPTANCE

Grace has experienced two very dissimilar spiritual awakenings. She was sitting in an AA meeting on one occasion and looked up to see a banner that read: "You are not alone." With sudden certainty, she knew this was true. She had a profound experience of connectedness and relief, and a heartwarming assurance that she was supported by the people around her and by life itself.

On another occasion she began crying about something so insignificant she doesn't even recall the problem. She let the tears flow for as long as they would come—"crying until the end of crying," as she says. "I cried for hours. It was as if all my bottled-up grief came to the surface." When she was done, she felt peaceful and cleansed. She came to an acceptance of all that had happened, and for all that would happen in the future. It was the beginning of her deep commitment to a spiritual life.

GRADUALLY EXPANDING AWARENESS

Norma considers each new realization in her recovery part of her spiritual awakening. It began when she admitted her powerlessness in Step One and continued as she came to believe in the existence of a power that would guide and support her. Norma's awakening grows deeper and stronger with each Step. Each letting go, each new insight into her feelings and behavior adds to it.

"The whole program is about creating greater awareness of my own experience," says Norma. "When I see how I connect with others and when I see what is getting in my way, my perspective grows larger. Each awareness contributes to my spiritual wholeness."

BLOSSOMING OF HOPE

Sometimes a spiritual awakening is symbolic, as Julia's was. Julia has many stories describing spiritual experiences through her fifteen years of sobriety, but a simple event moved her most deeply.

Julia had a special plant. In the ten years she had tended it in her apartment, it had never bloomed. At a time in her life when she felt utter despair about some serious difficulties, the plant began to bloom. Its small white flowers filled her apartment with their fragrance. It was a sign of hope and reassurance she needed. When the crisis was over, the blossoms faded. "I saw the blossoms as a sign there could be possibilities I hadn't yet imagined," says Julia.

PHYSICAL AWAKENING

Sometimes "awakening" is almost literal, particularly when we've been numb and shut down in our addictions. Darlene sensed that her *body* was finally awake. When she stopped eating compulsively, her awareness of her body changed. She experienced new feelings and sensations—new dimensions of her being. She no longer regarded her body as an enemy that humiliated her with its lack of control. Awakening from numbness and learning how her body felt was a spiritual awakening. "It was like coming back to life," she says.

This physical awakening is part of Darlene's deeper sense of spirituality, of self-discovery. The more fully she becomes who she is—physically, emotionally, and mentally—the more spiritually connected she feels. "Recovery and spirituality are about becoming who I am and learning that this true self is connected to everything else," she says.

WHAT NEXT?

Recovery isn't something we do in our spare time or only when we're in a crisis. Having had a spiritual awakening, we know our new way of thinking, feeling, and behaving is incompatible with using alcohol, drugs, money, food, or sex in an addictive way. It's self-destructive to go back to this kind of behavior knowing what we know now. We find that succumbing to our addiction is more stressful than ever once we are awakened to the alternative.

Still, relapse is always possible, and one of the ways we prevent it is to work with others. This is the active spirituality of Step Twelve. We "carry this message" so that others learn about the Steps and so that we continually remind ourselves of the basics of recovery. Whether our awakening comes overnight or over a period of years, we'll have something significant to share with another recovering woman: a sense of hope, acceptance, integrity, and wholeness. This is a powerful message to carry.

GIVING IT AWAY

By sharing our experiences with others we learn another of recovery's paradoxes: *we keep it by giving it away.*

Recovery is an experience of mutuality: we constantly give and receive. We become empowered by empowering others, and the way we do this is by sharing our experience, strength, and hope. This doesn't mean we "fix" others, give them advice, or do anything for them they can't do for themselves. It simply means we describe how our recovery has been for us. In the words of AA, we share "what we used to be like, what happened, and what we are like now."[1]

The simplest way to "Twelve Step" someone is to tell the stories of our drinking or using behavior, how we began recovery, and what our experience has been with the Steps. AA calls itself a program of "attraction, not promotion," which means people will be drawn into recovery and want to stay if they see we have something they desire—like sustained sobriety—but not if we try to sell them on the program. All we have to offer is our own story and the ability to empathize and listen to others.

Working with others doesn't apply only to newcomers who are struggling through their first thirty days of sobriety or abstinence; it means offering support to anyone who's in need of it. This could be someone who's been in the program for many years or someone who isn't in a program at all—a relative, a stranger, a co-worker— and is having a difficult time. The intention is to offer what we have to the person who is "still suffering." This could be anyone, anywhere.

How we carry the message is completely up to us. We can be public or private in the way we share our experience of sobriety and abstinence. Sandy is open about her recovery in every aspect of her life, including the literature classes she teaches at a university. Her public disclosures have inspired at least two of her students to seek help for their drinking.

Many of us desire more privacy and anonymity, choosing to do most of our Twelve Step work within our recovery group. In many Twelve Step programs this means "service" and "sponsoring," but it can also mean simply being there when someone needs us or just showing up at meetings and listening.

Service involves helping a Twelve Step meeting run smoothly: setting up chairs, making coffee, ordering and setting out literature, collecting contributions, running the meeting, greeting newcomers, arranging for speakers. Many women find it comfortable and easy to take on service roles, all of which benefit the meeting and encourage us to show up consistently and get involved. Service can be a wonderful way to start to feel connected with a group while giving something back to it at the same time. Through service many of us begin to think how we might also serve our communities or other parts of the larger world.

Sponsoring means spending time with someone who may have less experience with the Steps and guiding her through. It's not about telling someone what to do or giving advice, but suggesting, observing, and sharing your own experience.

Being a sponsor is like being a "big sister" who helps another woman gain some perspective and sort through her feelings. But like everything else in recovery, sponsoring is a mutually helpful relationship. I've learned many things from the women I've worked with as a sponsor. Hearing about another woman's pain and watching her work through it has often been a mirror for my own experience, allowing me to gain a new perspective on my own feelings or memories.

CARING AND CARETAKING

Because women are expected to be giving, nurturing, and supportive, we need to take special care when we enter into Twelve Step work. It can be easy for us to slip into excessive caretaking and get so involved in others' recovery that we don't pay enough attention to our own. Just as common, we can use Twelve Step work to avoid our feelings.

At the end of her first year of sobriety, Eve was involved in a child-visitation battle with her ex-husband that caused her sleepless nights. No matter what kind of work she did with the Steps, she couldn't stop worrying. To help her "get out of her head," Eve's sponsor suggested she start sponsoring other women. "When all else fails, work with others," said her sponsor.

Eve put her name on a temporary sponsor list at a large meeting and soon got a call from Christine. When they met, Christine said she was still drinking and talked about a man she had met at her first meeting. After a few more conversations Christine stopped showing up at the AA group.

While her interaction with Christine distracted her for a while, Eve felt like a failure when it was over. Years later, she realizes that becoming a sponsor at that point in her sobriety was not wise. It wasn't helpful for her to focus on someone else. Now, instead of focusing outward when she feels unbalanced, she stays with her feelings. Instead of trying to help someone else, she asks for help for herself.

Eve's experience illustrates an important point: we must have something ourselves before we can give it away. Quite often women rush to assist others when they need help themselves. In AA this is called "two-stepping"—working the First and the Twelfth Step, but not the Steps between. A newcomer gets sober, admits her powerlessness, and immediately begins carrying the message to others. AA cautions against this because "obviously you cannot transmit something you haven't got."[2]

Instead, we want to make sure we're doing our part to maintain our sobriety and abstinence—exploring our faith, reviewing our past, identifying our patterns, learning how to let go of what we can't control, and engaging in life. This doesn't mean we must complete all of the previous Steps before we offer to support another person. But we do need to build a foundation if we're going to be helpful to anyone else.

Even when we have a strong foundation, we may find that we still need to guard against giving too much of ourselves away. Like Eve, Shannon was tempted to carry the message to someone who wasn't ready to hear it. While she was aware there was a limit to what she could do, she had to remind herself she couldn't control the outcome of the situation.

Shannon's brother is addicted to prescription drugs. Her first impulse was to send him a Big Book or take him to a meeting or at least give him a long lecture about the symptoms of addiction. She finally said, "Thomas, you have a serious problem with drugs. If you ever want help, I'm available to help you find it."

Thomas belligerently argued that he wasn't an addict and told Shannon to mind her own business. Shannon simply repeated herself: if he wanted help, she was available. She felt sad and relieved at the same time—sad that Thomas was being destroyed by his drug use and relieved that she had resisted the temptation to "fix" him. Thomas has never accepted her offer.

When we want to care for others, we must often make sure we're taking care of ourselves first. Sometimes recognizing our limitations can be one of the hardest things about supporting other people in recovery.

WALKING THE WALK

As we work the Steps we learn how to "talk the talk." We know the words and phrases common to recovery—First Things First, Turn

It Over, One Day at a Time, Keep It Simple. But it may take longer to "walk the walk"—to follow through on these suggestions. For instance, it may be easy to understand why "turning it over" is important, but harder to put the understanding into practice.

When we reach Step Twelve we're probably walking the walk more consistently each day. As the Twelfth Step says, we "practice these principles in all our affairs." We know the ideas of recovery and we try to *live* them.

By now we've had experience letting go, asking for help, and "owning" our patterns, habits, and behaviors. We are learning to turn inward to find a quiet place, to accept the things we cannot change, and to change the things we can.

This way of life has probably become more natural over time. You may be surprised to realize you prefer to act in these ways rather than going into denial, becoming isolated, and struggling to change things beyond your control. This new way of being is a spiritual awakening. What a miracle to participate in life this way! Practicing these principles leads to the gift of a more balanced and joyous life.

When faced with a crisis you might find yourself naturally turning to your new principles to sustain you. You may discover that the basics of the Twelve Step program work just as well with your daily challenges as they did with your drinking or using.

When Julia's husband told her about his affair with a younger woman and asked for a divorce, she felt emotionally overwhelmed. Many old, self-destructive feelings came up: "I'm worthless, I'm unlovable, this is the end of the world." But Julia quickly remembered a fundamental recovery wisdom: *One Day at a Time.* While she might feel wretched today, the feeling wouldn't last forever, and she knows she can find support to handle the pain.

"Staying in today" doesn't remove Julia's pain, but it does prevent her from panicking, believing she'll be miserable the rest of her life. She knows some new opportunity will arise from this upheaval—not necessarily reconciliation, but some valuable and worthwhile lesson. She has faith that things will change and that she will change too.

When we walk through pain like this and use the principles of the program to help us navigate and even grow through it, we are walking the walk. We become living proof of the power of the Steps and the healing nature of recovery.

By simply taking care of ourselves, we carry the message of recovery. People notice when we greet life's ups and downs with centeredness and integrity. We demonstrate with our actions that it's possible to regain our balance even when life throws us a curve.

Women rely on the program to help them through illness, bankruptcy, a jail sentence, the death of a loved one, and even to face their own death. A woman who developed AIDS in her ninth year of sobriety surrounded herself with friends from her AA group. As she drew closer to death, they grieved together and supported each other. Each friend was touched by her strength and learned from her courage, and she, in turn, was comforted by their presence.

When we see women use the principles of recovery for the ordinary stresses of everyday life—the child care hassles, the fender benders, the bounced checks, the marital spats—we see their healing power in action.

A RECIPE FOR CHANGE

No matter how you carry the message, remember that you aren't obliged to sell recovery to anyone else (it doesn't work anyway) or to think of yourself as a representative of a particular Twelve Step program. Instead, you can be genuine and give what you have to give: your experience, strength, and hope. You may want to communicate the basics of the program as well as your individual perspective.

Maureen thinks of carrying the message as sharing a recipe with a friend. "When you get a recipe you like," she says, "you might start to modify it, adding a little something here and taking away something else there. Eventually the combination of ingredients suits your tastes.

"But when you give the directions to your friend, you might wonder if she'll like your personalized version of the recipe. Perhaps she'd like the original better. Or maybe she'll want to create her own individual variation, just as you did." So Maureen suggests giving both versions to your friend.

With recovery this can mean that we offer a straightforward explanation of the Twelve Steps as well as our own personal experience—how we reworked, translated, revised, or otherwise molded the Steps until they were relevant to us.

We all have more to offer than the party line and a by-the-book recitation of the Steps. We can share our story any way we like. As long as we're honest and sincere, we can't go wrong. It's as simple as saying, "This worked for me and it might work for you too."

Something amazing happens when we share ourselves: when we hear ourselves describe our recovery experience, we see how far

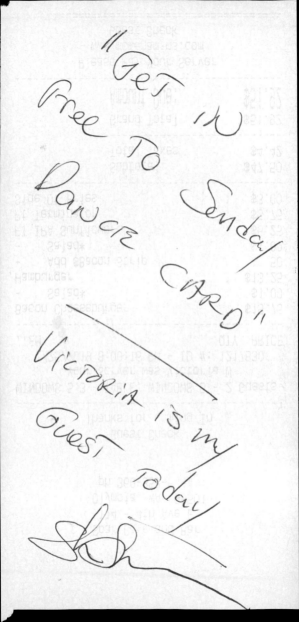

"GET IN
Free TO Sunday/
TO Dance CARD"

VICTORIA is my
Guest Today/

Spar Cafe and Bar
114 - 4th Ave E.
Olympia, WA 98501
ph 360-357-6

Guest Check
Thanks for Coming In

WINDOWS 5:3 - TABLE: WINDOWS 5 - 2 Guests
Your Server was Victoria W
7/25/2019 8:00:16 PM - ID #: 1217830

ITEM	QTY	PRICE
Bacon Cheeseburger	1	$15.75
- Salad*		$1.00
Hamburger	1	$13.25
- Add $Bacon Strip		50
- Salad*		$1.00
PT IPA Sunflower		$6.25
Pt Terminator		$5.75
Side Of Fries	1	$3.00

Subtotal		$47.50
Total Taxes		$4.42
Grand Total		$51.92
Amount Due:		**$51.92**

Please Pay Your Server
www.mcmenamins.com
Guest Check

we've come. For most of us it's been a long, miraculous journey from Step One to Step Twelve. We feel a profound gratitude when we share our recovery story with someone else. It gives us a chance to appreciate the new way of life we have—how *alive, present,* and *aware* we've become.

In telling our story, we may see more deeply into ourselves. Sometimes we don't know who we are or how we got from there to here until we describe our journey to someone else. So our sharing continues the upward spiral. We gain more by giving it away. In the mutually supportive environment of recovery, we depend on others as they depend on us, to constantly grow and evolve, to become our genuine selves. Having had a spiritual awakening, we become integrated and whole. We find new direction in our lives and the joy of balanced and purposeful living.

A Step After

W<small>E FIRST USE THE</small> T<small>WELVE</small> S<small>TEPS</small> to recover from addiction—to stop drinking or using. But as we look back, we find that the Steps have created a foundation upon which we can build our lives.

Before recovery, many of us never had a guide to turn to when our lives became difficult. After working the Twelve Steps to heal from addiction, we discover we can take what we have learned and apply it to something beyond drinking or using. Having developed the inner resources to cope with our addiction allows us to change many other aspects of our lives in a way that we can *feel*.

The women who have shared their stories here say that they experienced this change most dramatically in four areas of their lives: self, relationship, sexuality, and spirituality. These four areas are powerful indicators of the growth and expansion that can happen in recovery. They are also areas that may trigger a relapse. But these issues do not need to be stumbling blocks. They are the areas of life that give real depth and meaning to recovery.

Women who used to face problems in any one of these areas by drinking or using now talk about being surprised at how they can cope with difficult situations or stresses in life. In the course of recovery, they find tools for dealing with feelings and situations that used to overwhelm them, leave them nonfunctional, or drive them to drink or use again. They find an inner strength and a sense of knowing what each needs to do for herself.

Working with the Twelve Steps from a woman's perspective empowers us and helps us change our lives. Creating a strong inner place and believing there is something in the universe supporting us helps us to know we are not alone. Then we may be surprised to find that the power and healing revealed in the Steps allows an ease in living, an acceptance and serenity, that can transform the way we experience self, relationship, sexuality, and spirituality—which are at the heart of life.

Self

BEGINNING RECOVERY IS ABOUT DISCOVERING the self. When we come into recovery we expect to focus on alcohol or drugs or food or sex or money, or some combination of these that was our addictive behavior. Recovery is about addiction, but it is about much more: it is about finding out who you are and coming to a deeper understanding of your self.

The self is what is unique about our identity and character. It helps us organize our experience and make sense of our reality. The self gives purpose and direction to our choices and behavior. It is the part of us that says I feel, I like, I want, I know.

When we were addicted, our connection to our self—our experience, our feelings, and our deep inner knowing—was cut off. We were numbed, confused, unclear, and disconnected. We had lost our capacity to know what was true for our self, and without that sense of self, we lost our ability to relate with others.

"I had totally lost my self in my addiction," says Marta. "And losing my self, I didn't know what I wanted, what I felt, or what to do next. I was unconscious, codependent, and disconnected, and that's how I experienced myself in relationship—not only to myself but to the universe and to everything in it."

We first begin to discover ourselves in recovery by acknowledging our addiction. This is a paradox of recovery: we begin to heal ourselves by first identifying with the addiction that has damaged the self. When we go to meetings, we introduce ourselves with, "Hello, my name is _____. I am an alcoholic." This first identification with our addiction helps us begin the process of looking at self. Later, as our recovery continues, we find that this identification is only one aspect of self.

"For the first three or four years in recovery I identified myself as an alcoholic. I wore that as my badge—that was who I was, and that was really all I could be. Today I'm Maureen, and I happen to have a disease, but that's not where I started," says Maureen.

Identifying honestly with our addiction may be our first opportunity to think about ourselves, to ask the question, Who am I? This question leads us to a deeper understanding of the self—to what is changeless and unique about each of us.

"Before coming into recovery I thought there was no self," said Darlene. "I'd been numbed and medicated. Looking in the mirror became impossible. Either I didn't want to see who was there, or I didn't want to know that there wasn't anyone. It was frightening not having a self I knew. Asking, Who am I? and defining myself as a separate entity with a unique identity was the next big piece of my recovery."

To start to discover your unique identity you might begin to make a list of words that describe who you are. Leave out words like *mother* and *wife,* or job titles. These words describe some of the roles you play, but not *who* you are.

You might find you struggle with this exercise and don't have anything to list. It may be hard to come up with words to describe who you *are* rather than what you *do.* Try working with your sponsor or a friend. Ask trusted people around you to suggest words to help fill out your picture of yourself. You will find this process urges you to go deeper inward to ask yourself, Who am I? What words describe what is unique about me?

As your Twelve Step journey continues, your sense of self, your picture of who you are, is likely to change. Keep working on your list over the course of your recovery and see how your picture of yourself grows and changes. You will probably find you move from your first self-identification with your addiction to a deeper, more complex sense of who you are.

This more complex sense of self includes the feelings unique to each of us. So, our second question is, What do I feel?

Recognizing our feelings can be a frightening process. For years we avoided feelings through our addiction. We numbed ourselves with alcohol or drugs or food or a whole variety of other addictive behaviors. We disconnected our thoughts from our feelings so that we would not know what we were feeling; in fact we didn't really *feel* at all. It was as if we were in a perpetual fog. We were disconnected from our feelings, with little sense of an inner life.

When we stopped our addictive behaviors, we were often surprised by the strength of our feelings. Many women in early recovery talk about being overwhelmed by feelings. "Before recovery, I was numb. I didn't know what I felt or who I was," says Constance. "With sobriety came a flood of feelings, and eventually I came to recognize and use parts of myself—talents and strengths—I never knew I had."

I, too, experienced this confusion of feelings after I got sober. When I began to have feelings, I had no idea what they were. All I knew was that I *felt*. "Oh my God, I'm feeling . . . what is it?" I wondered. I didn't have a clue.

At first you may experience only a vague sensation. You may not even have words to describe it. Often it is helpful to look at a list of feeling words. As you begin to sort out your feelings and put language to vague sensations, you come closer to finding out who you really are.

Although what we feel isn't *who* we are, recognizing our feelings is part of the journey towards discovering our self. As we move deeper into our self, we find that we are able to clarify what we feel. Exploring these feelings leads to an undiscovered inner reality that eventually reveals more about the self.

Once we begin to recognize and identify our feelings, we then begin to ask ourselves a third question: What do I like, or what do I want? By examining our values, we begin to match our inner feelings with our outer behaviors.

When we were addicted, we often found ourselves acting against our own value systems. Many of us said, "I won't be drunk at my son's wedding," but we were; or "I'd never consider having an affair," but we did; or "I would certainly never binge on chocolate cake in a public place," yet we ate piece after piece. Each time we did something contrary to our values, we suffered a loss of self and a lowered sense of self-esteem.

"Breaking my value system in my addiction played on my shame," said Darlene. "I'd tell myself, 'I'll never drive drunk when I pick the kids up after school,' and then I would. That triggered my core sense of being unworthy, and then I wanted to move out of relationship. I wanted to hide and break the very connections that meant the most to me."

When we begin to recognize our feelings as a signal that we don't like something we're doing, we reconnect our inner reality with our values. This is a process of expanding our feeling self. Being able to feel on a much broader spectrum with a lot more subtlety empowers us to grow and become whole. Understanding that we have an inner self and an outer self allows us to expand our sense of self. Then we can connect the inner and the outer self, matching our feelings, our values, and our needs to our choices and our behaviors. But we have to be in touch with our inner reality, to first know *what* we are feeling.

What do I feel? What do I need? What do I want? Most women struggle with the answers to these questions because we were trained to put others and relationships first: what does he want, what do they need, what does she like? Often the very act of examining our own needs and desires becomes lost in our efforts to respond to others.

Even if we ask these questions of ourselves, we often adjust our answers to fit the expectations of others. Many of us learned to define ourselves in terms of our roles: I am someone's daughter, someone's lover, someone's wife. We learned to look to someone else to tell us how we were performing these roles, to tell us we were "good enough." In looking to others, we hid what we felt and desired in order to gain acceptance. Eventually we lost touch with our feelings and desires and separated our inner self from our outer life.

This culturally ingrained pattern of separating from self is complicated by addiction. Addiction can be described as the continuing neglect of self in favor of something or someone else. In fact, when we become addicted to something, we habitually neglect ourselves—who we are and what we need.

Many of us found it especially difficult to maintain a sense of self in relationships. We drank or used drugs when we found our relationships hurtful, unfulfilling, or abusive. We may have joined our partners in alcohol or drug use so that we had some sense of connection, however slender. We may have tried many addictive ways to change ourselves to fit the relationships available, only to find we had lost our self-esteem and our sense of self.

Jackie, a compulsive spender, used money to try to hold on to relationships. "I came into the Twelve Step program through compulsive debt, and that tied into my sense of myself," she says. "I would spend compulsively, ignoring the connection between my outgo and my income, usually because there was something I felt I had to have or do in order to make myself more acceptable to other people, specifically men. I was trying to enhance my self-esteem, to make myself less likely to be abandoned."

We may think our addictions are building our sense of self by keeping us connected in relationships. They are, in fact, self-destructive. "I lost myself in my addiction and with people," continues Jackie. "I was confused about what I felt, and I put myself at risk. I was chronically depressed and living on the edge as a way to keep feeling alive and connected."

Alcohol, drugs, sex, or spending didn't help us make or keep the connections that kept us alive and related, they isolated us further. Almost all addicted women talk about isolation and alienation. As our lives became more and more focused on our addiction, we became more limited by its demands.

Recovery is about expansion. The Twelve Step path is an ever-widening spiral. At first we circle tightly around our addiction, then, as we begin our recovery, our lives begin to expand. The object of addiction no longer binds us so tightly. We begin to include more experiences and more people in our lives. This is the process of expanding the self.

We begin to expand the self by going to our first Twelve Step meeting. First we identify ourselves with our addiction and admit our powerlessness over it. Next we begin to expand our perception of ourselves by sharing our experience and hearing it echoed in a Twelve Step group. We expand our environment, our world, and our shared experience.

When we were isolated, when life was about walking out the front door to the liquor store and getting a bottle and coming home, our worldview and our sense of self were very narrow and confined. The more things we do and the more people we include in our lives, the more our world and our experience of self can expand. When we are connected with more people, we have a greater capacity for seeing ourselves in different experiences.

Through these experiences we eventually come to know and name our values, wants, needs, and feelings. We get to know who we are apart from our addictions and the roles we play. Our recovery is a process of becoming whole, or complete, by asking questions and learning about and naming the self in new and different ways.

It is through this process of recovery that our sense of self begins to emerge. As Sandy says, "Recovery is when you look inside and begin to ask, What do I think? What do I feel? What is my truth? What are my options? Then you can start resonating inside yourself and figuring out what is true for you—not what will please other people or make them happy. We literally need to give birth to the self."

The spiritual path of the Twelve Steps leads us toward self-recognition and redefinition. In Step One, we surrender to an honest identification with our addiction that helps us to name ourselves. In Steps Two and Three we find that surrender brings us to a deeper, wiser Self, the Higher Power, however we define it. This allows us to accept a new, deeper self-definition. Our self expands from a one-dimensional addicted self to a multifaceted self in relationship to others and to God as we understand him or her.

Steps Four, Five, Six, and Seven are all about getting to know ourselves. We continue to expand the self when we choose to name and clarify our self-defeating behaviors and to identify what is good about us.

Julia knows how important it is for women to see what is good in themselves. "Many women are all too ready to leap into a searching and fearless moral inventory with harsh judgment, looking only for negatives," she says. "As women we are constantly told about our defects of character, so we're very good at acknowledging our defects. We don't often hold other people accountable yet will hold ourselves overaccountable, taking all the responsibility and blame upon ourselves. All our lives we've been judging ourselves and finding out what is wrong. It is hard for us to say what's good about ourselves, what our assets are. A key piece of rediscovering our selves is also to name what is good about us."

Sandy agrees that the Steps are about acknowledging the good intentions underlying our "defects" and shortcomings. "Step Five, admitting our 'wrongs,' must include, for women, an admission of our strengths—our talents, our beauty, our wisdom, as well. All of these come from our Creator and are to be celebrated," she says.

When we identify ourselves with our strengths, we begin to grow and flourish. Then we can start to discover and define the self in expanded ways in relationship. Our experiences of being connected to others in new, healthy ways leads to expanded ideas about self.

The path has brought us full circle again to relationship. But we notice with surprise that we are not in the same place we started. This time we do not identify ourselves only by our addictions or by our roles.

Gradually, we reclaim what is rightfully ours. "Now I have a deeper sense of myself," says Darlene. "I have an essence that I have reclaimed, and along with the reclaiming of my essence, my self, I have discovered the courage to redesign myself and become who I am today. I had to be abstinent to do that, and I couldn't do it alone. I needed guidance and support."

Following the Twelve Step path leads us to a deeper sense of our self. But what do we do when we get there?

"Walking the path is necessary to finding our self. But I say that self without relationship, like faith without works, is dead," says Katy. "There is, in reality, no such thing as working on feeling good about myself to simply find myself. My true sense of self comes from works, from action, from right relationship."

Identifying ourselves by our addiction opens the door to an unexplored inner reality where we first discover the self. This self expands as we identify the attributes and feelings that are unique to us. We cultivate a profound reconnection to self, to our values, and to life-giving relationships. We begin to live from the inside out rather than from the outside in.

"We are in a sense diverted off our own path," says Grace. "But recovery is coming back to ourselves, to our strengths, to our way of knowing and being in the universe. Being restored to sanity means being restored to our deepest selves."

Relationship

As we learn to be true to ourselves—to know our feelings, needs, and values—we bring this inner knowing to our relationships with others. In recovery, we begin to make better choices about our relationships, and we learn to create relationships based on mutual caring as well as self-care.

The relationships we create during recovery are the container in which we do our healing work. We find others in recovery who are willing to listen without criticism or judgment and who share their experiences so that we feel connected and assured that we are not alone in our struggles.

Just as an infant needs a safe, nurturing environment to grow and develop, so do we. We all need a place where we feel safe, loved, cared for, and understood. It is in this environment that we heal.

Relationships are the soil that nourishes our lives. We are who we are in relation to other people: our partners, children, employers, co-workers, neighbors, friends, and family. All these connections give us a sense of self and self-worth.

In fact, women tend to establish their identity in relation to other people. This doesn't mean that we derive our identity *from* other people, but that *we have the capacity to discover our potential for authenticity, competence, and wholeness within our relationships.*

Under the best circumstances, we prosper and grow as a result of our meaningful connections with other human beings. "Women tend to find satisfaction, pleasure, effectiveness, and a sense of worth if they experience their life activities as arising from and leading back into a sense of connection with others," says Dr. Jean Baker Miller.[1]

This desire to be connected to others can be life affirming and healthy. But when we are in nonaffirming or abusive relationships, this desire becomes distorted and causes harm and pain.

"The basic issue for women is relationships," says Shannon. "But you know, I think many women have been or are in relationships that have been hurtful and harmful and painful."

Many of us didn't grow up under the best circumstances. We may have experienced physical or sexual abuse in our families or early lives. Or our families may have been emotionally incapable of giving us the love, security, and sense of worth we needed. Our adult relationships may have been equally empty or abusive. These violations or disconnections can leave a void.

Like Shirley, some women used alcohol and other drugs to fill the void of what was missing from early relationships. "My father drank, sometimes heavily, and when he drank, he raged and beat me. Early on I felt this continuous struggle to feel good about myself—to feel valued and to make my parents proud of me," says Shirley. "That was my basic need. I felt unvalued, and I felt this emptiness inside me, so I drank."

Sometimes we got into an addiction to make and maintain connections. We might have been in a relationship with an addict and believed the way to make or keep the connection with our partner was to use alcohol or drugs as he or she did.

"My boyfriend would go out drinking every night," says Natalie. "I couldn't get him to do anything with me, and I felt lonely and abandoned. Finally I decided that if he wouldn't do things with me, at least I could go and drink with him."

At some point, we begin to realize that the addiction didn't fill the emptiness, take away the reality, or make or keep the connections that we desired. The addiction, along with our diminished self-esteem, kept us locked into relationships that destroyed, rather than nourished our sense of self. We continued to feel disconnected, disempowered, unclear, confused, and worthless.

For some women this sense of confusion and disconnection may have lead to even greater alienation and isolation. Julia thought of herself during her drinking years as an "alien," as if she were on the wrong planet. It seemed to her that everyone else knew how to think, act, feel, and respond to life, but she didn't have a clue, and she hated herself for her inadequacy. She brought this battered self-esteem into her relationships, which led to even more desperation and unhappiness.

"When you hate yourself, you give people enormous power over you," says Julia. "All my relationships were distorted and imbalanced. I could only begin to have whole relationships when I had a sense of wholeness within myself."

Like many women who found their sense of worthlessness and inadequacy too painful to bear, Lois decided that she just wanted to be left alone. "I didn't like myself, and so I didn't like anyone else," she says. "I just didn't have the energy for human interaction."

There is another way in which our addiction distorted or disconnected us from our relationships: it created a triangle in each of our relationships. When our addiction competed for attention, we made choices that hurt our relationships.

Darlene's addiction directly interfered with her ability to relate to her children and to be the kind of parent she wanted to be. "I was completely self-absorbed, with no capacity for connection," Darlene recalls. "As a mother, I was critical, demanding, immature, self-involved, and emotionally unavailable—so bottom line, a really bad mother. The addiction came first."

Even our relationships themselves may have become addictive. We may have become so enmeshed in our relationships—like Natalie who "shared" her addiction with her partner, or like others who sought to fill an increasing sense of emptiness that substances could not fill—that we lost our own identity. We became intensely focused on "protecting our supply" or avoiding "withdrawal" from the attention, sex, status, companionship, or whatever else we received from the relationship.

This sense of desperation—Why hasn't he called? Is she thinking about me? How can I be more pleasing, more likely to get what I want?—does not allow for genuine relationships, for true intimacy and mutual caring.

As long as we stayed in a self-shaming state, disconnected from our true value and worthiness, we continued to seek relationships that gave us the same message that we gave ourselves: that we're hopeless, inept, and lacking in some elusive quality that everyone else seems to have. It was a vicious circle that ended with our journey through the Steps.

The source of our suffering and often of our addiction was in our attachments, the relationships in which we hoped to find satisfaction and a sense of worth. But it is one of the paradoxes of recovery that while our relationships caused us pain and suffering, our relationships are also going to heal us.

Early in recovery, it may be difficult to discover ways of developing in connection with others without agreeing to things that are hurtful. In the past, being in relationship meant giving up our needs and hiding our feelings to meet another person's needs, or changing ourselves to keep the relationship. When we talk about our growing, flourishing self and its development in relationship, we are talking about our self-development in healthy relationships of all kinds.

"I see the self as the way of being in a relationship," says Grace, "and I am talking about all kinds of relationships, not just primary relationships or sexual relationships. It's relationship between parent and child, it's relationship between siblings, it's relationship with grandmother and grandfather, it's relationship to the woman next door, it's relationship with your employer. It is all these ways of connecting with other human beings that give us a sense of self and self-worth."

We don't recover in isolation. We heal in relationship and in connection with other people. In recovery we move from isolation to connection.

Think about what happens in Twelve Step meetings. We come in addicted and alone and find that others share our experience; we can ask for and get help; we can speak our truth and hear others speak theirs; we can be vulnerable and still feel safe and protected.

"Early in my recovery I was engrossed in the pain and the stark fear of my surroundings—my relationship, the beatings, the alcohol," says Shirley. "But the nurturing spirit of the meetings and the encouragement not to drink got me out. It was in the acceptance and the belongingness and the fellowship of the meetings that I got out of that relationship and out of my addiction."

Our family relationships, friendships, and love relationships may have been abusive, disconnected, and isolating. They may have contributed to our addictive behavior. But in recovery, we begin to make healthy connections—connections that are "mutual, creative, energy-releasing, and empowering for all participants."[2]

"Until I began to recover, I never allowed myself to be around the kind of people I respected—people who were creative and successful in their inner as well as outer lives," says Jackie. "I had an 'addiction' to deprivation, and I wouldn't allow myself to have gratifying relationships. Gradually, I've become able to accept more and more gratification, and the quality of my relationships has increased. The people I allow myself to hang out with are fun to be with, offer me love and support, and encourage and stimulate my creative efforts."

It is in working the Steps *in relation to others* that we begin to heal ourselves and our relationships. In Step Two we open ourselves to a connection with a Power greater than ourselves that offers healing and support. We begin to feel less alone and alien as we become aware that we don't have to heal by ourselves.

Steps Four and Five provide a mirror in which we see ourselves reflected and allow ourselves to be seen. We can start to see ourselves with compassion when we begin to understand how our pain has caused us to build the defenses—or defects—we used to protect ourselves. When a sponsor or trusted friend listens to our story and accepts us as we are, we learn to look at ourselves and our behavior objectively and without judgment.

The first time Shirley did Step Four, she could only see the hurt and pain of her past. "Down the road, as I got on with understanding, I did another Fourth Step," says Shirley. "I made a conscious effort to look at where I had participated in the things going on in my life. I saw that I had lied, cheated, stolen, manipulated, conned, beaten, bullied, been aggressive—I mean, what a list! I could simply own the behaviors, not judge whether I was right or wrong. With the nurturing and the validation I got, I could see which part needed healing and which needed changing."

In making a direct connection with another person in Step Five, we learn what happens when we allow ourselves to be "seen." By sharing our stories, we allow another to experience and accept us as we are. This becomes a model for other relationships—for giving and receiving acceptance. We learn how to take the risk of being genuine and open, of speaking aloud our inner truth.

Relationships help us heal and change. They help us do the inner work to develop an authentic relationship with ourselves that is necessary to making healthy connections in the outer world.

Before we can make healthy connections, we may need to let go of the destructive relationships we stayed in because we wanted love and affirmation, because we were afraid we couldn't make it on our own, or because we were afraid there wouldn't be anything better. We may also want to let go of relationships based on past alcohol and drug use.

There's another kind of letting go. We may need to learn to be less controlling of our relationships. Now that we're in recovery, we may want our significant others to be in recovery too. Like Shannon, whose brother is addicted to prescription drugs, our first impulse may be to send a friend, partner, or family member a Big Book, take him or her to a meeting, or lecture about the symptoms of addiction. Remember, Twelve Step programs are based on attraction, not promotion. Often all we can do is live our lives as an example and let go—letting others find their own way in their own time.

We may also need to learn an emotional letting go. How do we keep from reacting when others respond negatively, or not at all, to the changes in us? Staying centered in our own program and working the Steps helps us keep our focus on ourselves. Then we can begin to develop new relationships and new ways of interacting in old relationships.

As we work the Steps, we being to practice self-acceptance and, by extension, the acceptance of others. When we stop judging ourselves harshly, we begin to judge others less harshly as well. This opens the door to more loving, honest relationships. We become more receptive to what others are experiencing without losing sight of what we are experiencing ourselves.

As we accept ourselves and others, as we let go of destructive relationships, of control, of emotional attachment, we develop our capacity for authentic and intimate relationships with ourselves and others. We begin to love with detachment. Detachment means "seeing reality as it is, not as your dreams would like it to be. It means letting go of rigidly held plans, assumptions, and expectations. Finally it means disentangling your personal boundaries from those of another person, getting a clearer sense of where your limits are or need to be."[3]

As we develop a clearer sense of ourselves and others, we move into Steps Eight and Nine. In making amends, we look at how our behavior contributed (or contributes) to our problems in relationships. We do not simply apologize; we live our amends by being responsible and responsive to ourselves and others. As Marta says, "In every situation, I now respond, rather than react. That means taking the time to think a situation through and make a decision about the best possible response."

This is our recovering self in relationship. The Steps invite us to pause and reevaluate the meaning of relationship and to learn how we can establish healthy connections with others in relation to our growing, expanding self.

Recovery requires expansion. Through the Steps we create and cultivate an inner life—a sense of our values, feelings, and beliefs. Then we integrate our inner life with our outer life—our actions with other people in the world. Recovery gives us a chance to make better choices about relationships: we can choose to enter into and sustain healthy relationships.

How will we know a healthy relationship when we see one? First of all, a healthy relationship is an honest relationship. In a healthy relationship, we can be true to ourselves and true to the other.

"Today, because I love myself enough, I put my best self forward by being honest with myself—with what's really going on with me. 'To thine own self be true,' " says Jackie. "I try to do this in all my relationships. When I compromise, it's almost like 'soft' prostitution—there's something I'm trying to get, and that's a form of manipulation. What I need to do is be direct and honest about what's going on with me and let other people deal with it as they choose."

A healthy relationship is an equal relationship. Equality means neither person is dependent on the other to give them something they feel they are missing.

"I am a full-fledged, capable human being first, and on equal terms in a relationship," says Sandy. "Early in my recovery I didn't feel capable, and I did some leaning-on in relationships. I let myself be taken care of emotionally and physically."

Equal relationships exist when both partners are free to give and take without using power over the other to feel secure. Sandy continues, "The less leaning I do, the more direct I can be. And when I'm direct about what I want and need, that takes the power imbalance out of the relationship. Recovery has taught me that being direct and honest works best in all instances."

A healthy relationship is one in which each person is free to know and be known without fear of manipulation or betrayal. Each of us can reveal our inner self and trust the other to honor and respect our experience and feelings.

Empathy, sensitivity to and understanding of another's experience, is another element in a healthy relationship. The ability to appreciate another person's experience is the cornerstone of fulfilling relationships. Empathy is the ability to join with another person at both a thinking and feeling level without losing connection to our own thoughts and feelings.[4]

Julia is developing her empathy through the "authenticity" she experiences in her relationships in recovery. "The people who love me, love me for the qualities I value in myself," she says. "They understand and love me knowing full well my weaknesses, my defenses, my vulnerabilities. As a result, I have a lot of tolerance for people—people who are different from me, people who have had different experiences."

There are other qualities in healthy relationships, or what Miller calls "growth-fostering" relationships:

- A *sense of increased zest or vitality*—meaning that everyone involved feels energized and alive in the relationship
- *Empowerment to act*—meaning there is freedom to make choices about the relationship and act on them
- *Knowledge of self and the other person*—which grows out of the interaction and exploration made possible by an environment of acceptance
- *A greater sense of self-worth*—which both of you experience by being able to communicate your true feelings
- *A desire for more connection*—with each other and with other people, to expand the experience of self-discovery.[5]

Many of us may experience these qualities of relationship for the first time in recovery. Getting to know ourselves and allowing others to know us creates an excitement about the possibilities for relationship. Connecting ourselves to a Higher Power and to others in recovery expands our experience of self, increases our sense of self-worth, and empowers us to act in healthy ways.

Recognizing, choosing, and maintaining growth-fostering or healthy relationships is the first step on the journey toward intimacy. When we think of intimacy, we may first connect it with sexual relationships. But intimacy has a place in other relationships too—in friendships and family relationships. Intimacy takes place in any relationship where we are willing to let ourselves be seen and known. It happens when we are open and vulnerable and willing to share our innermost self.

An authentic, intimate relationship is mutual: "Each person can represent her feelings, thoughts, perceptions . . . and can *move with* and *be moved* by the feelings of the other. Mutual influence, mutual impact, and mutual responsiveness characterize such relationships."[6]

Ruth, whose friendships when she was drinking were inauthentic and empty, says, "Now in my sobriety I'm aware of who my closest, most intimate friends are. I have wonderful relationships, characterized by a mutual commitment to growth and change and honesty."

In a mature, intimate relationship we also experience reciprocity —a shared interest in giving and receiving, while staying connected to our self. Dr. Janet L. Surrey describes this reciprocity:

> *It becomes as important to understand as to be understood, to empower as well as be empowered. . . . All of us probably feel the need to feel understood or "recognized" by others. . . . women all through their lives feel the need to "understand" the other—indeed desire this as an essential part of their own growth and development, as an essential part of self-worth.*[7]

In a reciprocal relationship, we share a common desire to create and maintain the relationship. We both find the relationship valuable and put equal energy into being together and to listening and supporting each other. Both feel equally able to be vulnerable and to trust.

Elena describes this reciprocity in the relationships she is developing in recovery. "I feel very connected and less afraid of expressing how I feel and letting my good friends know how important they are to me," she says. "I'm much more open now in terms of being able to reveal more about myself, and I'm more open to letting my good friends reveal more about themselves to me."

To create mutual commitment and reciprocity in an intimate relationship, we must first do the inner work. In recovery we begin developing a healthy self—one who knows who she is and what she feels and wants. To have an intimate relationship, it is important to allow what's happening on the inside to be reflected accurately in our outer life. When there is a discrepancy between our inner and our outer life, there is no foundation for trust, and intimacy is impossible. Intimacy depends on this authentic connection between the inner and the outer—what we feel, think, and want, and what we say and do.

When our inner and outer lives are in balance, we are open and free to know and be known. We are able to engage at a deep level with another—we are able to be intimate.

"It's only through recovery and the women I know that I can say, 'This is who I am, this is how I'm *feeling,*'" says Shirley. "There is validation and support when people say, 'Here, give me a call. Let's talk about it.' That heals, that brings about change, that bridges the gap."

When we bridge the gap, we sense that we are deeply connected by a dynamic, ceaseless flow of life. In the presence of another we can feel the creative current of energy that moves us toward expression and expansion through relationship.

So far we've looked at how we learn about and express emotional and intellectual intimacy in healing our relationships—how we express our feelings and thoughts in honest, empathic, mutually supportive, and reciprocal relationships. Physical intimacy, expressed through our sexuality, is also a part of the dynamic energy of healthy relationships we create in our recovery.

Sexuality

Being in recovery changes the way we experience our sexuality just as it changes the way we experience our self and our relationships. So during recovery it is important that we take the time to explore our sexuality.

We can't be whole and complete as women until we heal our sexual selves. We are all sexual beings. We need to embrace this life-giving part of ourselves if we are to accept ourselves completely and have the deepest possible relationships—with ourselves, with others, and with the sacred power that infuses our life.

During recovery we begin to reconnect to our sexuality by becoming aware of who we are as women, as sexual women, and as sexual women in relationship. Our sexual lives become more satisfying and fulfilling because they reflect our rediscovery of and appreciation for our inner life—our feelings, needs, and desires. As our recovery progresses, we learn to express this inner knowing and self-worth in our outer life—in our choices, our behaviors, and our connections with others.

The first step in healing our sexual selves is to understand that sexuality is more than sexual behavior, more than having sex (or not having sex). Our sexuality is a part of all aspects of our lives. Sexuality is not only physical, it is also emotional, psychological, and spiritual. It includes our perceptions, judgments, and feelings about ourselves and others, as well as how we act and with whom we act.

Like other aspects of our recovery, healing our sexual selves is a process that encompasses all of who we are and how we act in the world. As you will hear from other women in recovery, sexuality can be a yearning for connection that is alive, active, and whole-bodied. It may be a calling forth of the life force in our self and in another. Sexuality can be a doorway into and beyond the self—into relationship, into otherness. It can be the wellspring of ecstasy and the pathway to union with the sacred.

Healing our sexual selves depends on our being able to feel our sexuality from the inside. For many women, this inner sense of sexuality has been lost. We may not feel sexual, or if we do, we feel our sexuality in connection to some image or person outside of ourselves.

As we begin to explore our sexuality in recovery, we may wonder how sexuality can possibly be a life force within us when we have never connected to our sexual energy as a life-giving and self-affirming part of ourselves. In fact, sexuality may be the hardest and last place to heal because there are so many obstacles—inner and outer—to overcome.

There are many reasons we may have difficulty connecting with our own sexuality. Some of the obstacles to connecting with our sexuality come from cultural messages about what is "appropriate" or "desirable." Our past experiences, particularly if they were abusive or traumatic, also affected our sense of our sexuality. And our addictions affected our sexuality, as they did all other aspects of our lives, by breaking our connection with our self and others.

From early in childhood, we received messages from our families, churches, schools, and communities about our sexuality. Whether spoken or unspoken, many of those messages implied that "nice" girls aren't sexual. For many of us, this denial of our sexuality was compounded by our parents' confusion, embarrassment, or shame about sexuality, and we carried these feelings of confusion and shame into our adult lives.

Later, as adults, we may have allowed others, particularly our partners, to continue to define our sexuality. In our confusion and our disconnection from our sexuality, we looked to others to tell us what was pleasing, desirable, appropriate. This cut us off from our own inner experience—the ability to know, respond to, and ask for what pleases us.

Katy recalls the importance for her of being chosen and accepted by her partner. "I was very performance-oriented and very concerned about my desirability," she says. "I wanted to make sure that I was posed correctly and that I was accepted by the man. It was very important to be chosen as a sex object. But I wasn't really *there*."

Our feelings about our desirability also may have been influenced by the emphasis our culture puts on the importance of women's appearance. We have been bombarded by images of the ideal woman's size, shape, skin, hair, teeth, lips, thighs. Many of us have internalized this emphasis on the "perfect" appearance into negative feelings about our bodies. We feel pressured to conform to popular standards for beauty and appeal, and when we don't fit the outer images, we often feel ugly and undesirable on the inside.

The people closest to us may have knowingly or unknowingly reinforced these standards. Elena's mother bought her a girdle when she was in the fifth grade. This gave Elena a clear message that she needed to change her appearance to be acceptable. As a result, she says, "I always felt self-conscious about my weight and was never comfortable with myself physically."

When we cannot connect with our bodies in a positive and life-affirming way, our sexuality cannot flourish. Elena continues, "My sexuality was buried because I didn't feel comfortable being a woman and was afraid to be the person I am physically."

We may be disconnected from our sexuality in equally devastating ways when our sexual orientation is not validated. Because society and our families usually encourage or support only heterosexual relationships, an attraction we might have for another woman can provoke ridicule, anger, or denial. If our sexual identity has been challenged in this way, we may have felt ashamed or confused about our sexuality.

Shame and confusion also arise from past abuse. Any time there was sexual, physical, verbal, or emotional abuse in our past—whether we were molested or our bodies were the objects of jokes or obscene comments or leers—our sense of our sexuality was damaged.

There may be many of us who can identify with Shirley who says, "My first sexual experience was being raped." This violation of body and person at the most basic level deeply affects our perception of self and sexuality.

Because Shirley had been raped as a child and physically abused, she was ashamed of her sexuality and extremely fearful of sexual attention. She binged on food to make her body bigger, to hide her sexual self. "I used food to cover up my sexuality, to distance myself from my beauty, my energy, and my spirit," she recalls. "I just didn't want to draw attention to myself."

Alcoholism and other addictions are often linked with a history of abuse. Alcoholic women are more likely to have been abused—more frequently and for longer periods of time—than nonalcoholic women. And abused women are more likely to become alcoholic than those who have not been abused.[1] Our addictions may have been an attempt to erase these painful childhood memories, and while they may have worked temporarily, they also disconnected us from our adult sexuality.

When we compulsively used alcohol or cocaine, or even food or shopping, we lessened our connection with our sexual feelings and responses. We experienced the anxiety of craving and the numbness of using, which dulled our other sensations or physical experiences. Alcohol and other drugs actually suppress sexual response, making it difficult for us to respond to touch and become aroused.

Sex and addictions go hand in hand in other ways too. Some of us who are attracted to women found that we could act on our desire only if we were intoxicated. Some of us may have used alcohol or other drugs to loosen our inhibitions if we felt ashamed to act on feelings of sexual desire or even just express sensuality—to dance, to touch another person with affection, to enjoy how our bodies feel, to wear sexy clothing.

Some of us may have had sex to please another person and used alcohol, drugs, or food to numb ourselves to the reality that we were doing something we didn't want to do. Darlene recalls thinking this way about sexual relationships when she was drinking: "I thought I had to take whatever came my way, no matter how painful it was or whether I wanted it or not," she says. "If a man pressured me to have sex, I'd think, 'Oh, well. I'm drunk, and I don't want to piss him off.'" She didn't want to be sexual, but she was afraid of being physically injured if she resisted.

Shirley's relationship with her boyfriend was based on his being her drug supplier and her being his women. Perhaps we also used sexuality to get our drug of choice. Or maybe, as with Francesca, the sex simply came with the drinking. "I wasn't making a conscious choice," she says.

Many of us had never had a sexual experience apart from drinking or drug use. As Elena says, "I never had sex without drinking or doing a drug of some sort." But in recovery we begin to realize for the first time how our addictions have numbed and distorted our sexuality.

As we pay attention to our growing sense of self in recovery, we begin to sort out how our sexuality has been affected by outside influences—the messages we received from our families, churches, and the media. We examine the training, values, and prescriptions that no longer fit with our rediscovered inner self.

Through our sense of safety and connection with others in recovery, we begin to look at how our sexuality has been affected by our past experiences. For some women this means becoming aware of and healing the sexual abuse or trauma of the past. It is important for abuse survivors to seek a qualified therapist or support group to help heal this kind of trauma.

We also review our sexual behaviors and attitudes using the Twelve Steps to discover where we contributed to our disconnection from our sexuality and what we'd like to change about our sexual behavior.

It is sad to say that this might be difficult. The "no-talk" rule that our culture applies to topics of sexuality may also exist in

Twelve Step groups. Yet only when we begin to be aware of the old messages and experiences that distorted our sexuality and replace them with truth and understanding, can we begin to change.

When we begin to open up to our sexuality in sobriety, we may encounter sexual questions or problems. We may wonder if we will ever feel comfortable with our sexuality or safe and open with a sexual partner. It is helpful to talk with other women and learn they too have had similar experiences.

Relating her fears, Julia says, "In my drinking days I never made love when I was not drunk or hungover. When I got sober, I was afraid that I wouldn't be able to have sex without alcohol. I felt that alcohol liberated me, made me experimental, helped me do things I would otherwise not do."

Katy, who used sex to feel accepted and valued, says, "It was very important to me to be chosen as a sex object. I was afraid to face, sober, that I might not be admired and accepted by a man."

"I was molested. I was raped," says Shirley. "As I continued to recover, I had fears about how that would affect my sexual relationship with my husband."

For many of us, coming to know and value ourselves in recovery adds new dimensions and vitality to our old self-images. Julia says, "I was afraid when I stopped drinking that I would lose a part of myself that I valued—the risk-taker and experimenter. So it was important for me to do some sexual experimentation sober. I didn't want to feel I had to have alcohol in order to have access to that part of myself. So when I was sober, I actually did some bolder things sexually than I'd ever done drunk. And in some ways sex was even better, maybe because I had more safety—I knew what I was doing and I could choose."

Darlene, who could not recall ever having sex without being drunk, had to learn how to be sexual with her husband without alcohol. "I had this picture of myself as being this great siren because I had been so willing to 'service' men when I had been drinking," she recalls. "But now sex was suddenly real, and I was more interested in my own needs. We were present to each other and very aware. It was like being sixteen again. I had a real sense of wonder at the newness of it."

Reconnecting with our sexuality includes learning about or becoming reacquainted with our bodies—what we look like naked, what kinds of touch we respond to, when we feel sexual. It means looking at our bodies with curiosity and a willingness to embrace our particular expression of female beauty and sexuality. It means accepting ourselves as we are and caring for our bodies—for ourselves, rather than to please someone else.

"Now I feel very feminine when I get out of the tub and powder myself," says Lavonne. "I used to do that to please a man, but now I do it for me. I used to take care of my body hoping a man would see me and want me, but now I'm taking care of my body for my own pleasure and benefit."

We connect with our sexuality when we begin to believe we are desirable and beautiful in our own unique way. As Elena says, "My sexuality is feeling comfortable being a woman and not feeling afraid to be all the person I am physically."

Katy, who in the past used sex for acceptance, now finds that as she is getting to know herself in recovery, she is less concerned about her desirability. She finds that the admiration and acceptance she looked for from a man are available inside herself.

When we begin to feel comfortable with our inner sense of sexuality—our feelings, wants, needs, preferences—we then begin to connect them to outer actions and relationships.

When we live from the inside out, we may find our sexuality changes in ways we might not have thought possible. "I became much more sexually responsive," says Julia. "I became more orgasmic, more sensitive—I experienced all kinds of new sensations. It's true that it was awkward having sex with new people without alcohol—I'd never done it before! But it probably wasn't so great when I was drunk, either; I just didn't remember. Now I accept that the first time is always awkward. Everybody's nervous about performance, and whether this is a good idea, and is this the right person, and what's this going to be like, and so on. Now, sober, I'm conscious of all these questions, while in the past I was literally unconscious. So I feel I've had a much richer sex life sober than I ever did drunk. I am more able to ask for what I need, I'm more responsible, I'm more choosy. I'm also less inhibited in a strange way. I'm more open to different possibilities."

In recovery we learn to make choices about our feelings and behaviors in relation to others, and this extends to our sexual relationships. We can choose relationships where we can say yes or no and feel safe communicating our wants and needs with a partner who respectfully and lovingly responds.

Setting boundaries and then being able to set them aside by choice is essential to our sexuality. Shirley found that with the self-knowledge and self-acceptance she gained in her recovery, she was free to communicate her limits and boundaries with her husband. She says, "Now my sexuality means I enjoy sex to the fullest. I'm very expressive, I'm very comfortable, despite the fact I've been molested, despite the fact I've been raped. And honesty is the healing thing— to be able to say, 'This is how I'm feeling; this is not what I'm comfortable with.' I can now share that from the inside out."

Sexuality is not just about sex. Sexuality is often a yearning for mutuality and connection with another in a loving and caring relationship. This desire to feel close and be joined with a particular person is expressed in an urge to please and receive pleasure and to create a physical union.

As Jackie says, "Our sexual relationship is not just about sex. It's exciting in the way he responds to me, or the way he initiates things or I initiate something. It's exciting because I know we care about each other."

Our experience of our sexuality deepens in connection to another. When we take what we have learned about our inner selves and move outward toward a lover, we open ourselves to the possibility of joining in something greater than our separate self. As Dr. Judith V. Jordan notes, "[Sexuality] in the larger sense affirms our connection and being 'a part of' rather than 'apart from.' It leads to expansion rather than satisfaction; the former suggests growth, life, and openness; the latter suggests stasis."[2]

In recovery we develop a strong and healthy self—a woman who is comfortable with herself, who knows she is desirable and beautiful in her own way. This strong inner self then leads us to healthy and mature relationships. And it is within the depths of our selves and our relationships that we may also find the spiritual kinship described in *Awakening Your Sexuality:*

In sexual experience with an intimate partner, we may go beyond expressing our deep emotional involvement and erotic attraction; we may also touch each other's souls and express our spiritual affinity. In the act of sexual union with another, we can experience the wonderful loss of self that is akin to the mystical." [3]

"I actually do experience my life force as coming out of the yearning for connection," says Grace. "Somehow that energy is very sexualized. Just talking, I can go into this level of relating that feels very sexual—much more alive. I feel the blood flowing in all the parts of myself. It's alive, it's active, it's a whole-body experience. Sexuality gives a spiritual aliveness."

Sexuality does give a spiritual aliveness, and a power, that women are traditionally not supposed to have. Katy thinks that much of her drinking was to sublimate that power—the addiction was killing off the spirit. "But we rediscover God's power within when we are true to our own inner sensor," she says.

When we are true to this inner sensor, we can be open to a new freedom and new energy from within. We begin to sense our uniquely female body as the container of a life force greater than ourselves.

As Sandy says, "Sexuality is letting the spirit flow—letting the passion, the body, the energy get big, raucous, loud, powerful. It's about being alive, being you. It's really about connecting to your sense of inner power. When I feel it, I feel good on the inside."

Shirley relates to it this way: "I feel there is a strong source, a fountain running through me, coursing through me from an old wise woman that has been covered up by all this alcohol and other clamor. And the sexuality! When I'm making love I feel this surge of energy. I've come to the point of owning, claiming, and now flaunting my beauty, my energy, my spirit."

In the process of recovery this beauty, energy, and spirit come from within. This is our true sexuality. "And when that sexuality comes from within," says Grace, "just like with self and relationships, we shift from the pursuit of a high—a running after, trying to find ourselves or make connections, or trying to drink to be high—to a much more gentle, much more penetrating ability to stay with ourselves, with our source."

Finally our sexuality, like self and relationship, becomes more integrated. It ceases to be something outside, pushing us to do or feel or want, or compelling us to take what we think we need to survive. Instead, it comes from inside as a life force, an energy, a spirit connecting us to ourselves, to others, and to the sacred in our lives.

Spirituality

"ADDICTION BIRTHED MY SPIRITUALITY," Marta says. Spirituality can be a new dimension of life for women who've come into recovery. Birthing our spirituality in the recovery process opens us to all kinds of questions about spirituality. Who or what is this Power greater than ourselves? Can I trust it? What do I believe? What about church? What does it feel like to have a spiritual life? Am I spiritual?

If we hear the suggestion that we look inside to find our spirituality or our Higher Power, we may feel even more confused. Many of us don't feel a sense of spirituality inside when we first come into recovery. Instead we may feel numb or empty. We may not know there's anything inside us at all. We may wonder why and ask, Am I really empty? Is there anything that can fill me? Can love do that? Can another person do that? Can God or a Higher Power?

It is often said that addiction, whether to alcohol, drugs, food, or sex, is one way we try to fill the emptiness we feel inside. Of course it doesn't work: the emptiness returns as soon as we stop drinking or using. But this search for something to fill the emptiness gives us a clue about spirituality.

Carl Jung, writing in response to a letter from Bill Wilson said, "Alcohol in Latin is *spiritus* and you use the same word for the highest religious experience as well as for the most depraving poison.

The helpful formula therefore is: *spiritus contra spiritum*[1]—the spirit against spirits.

When we stop trying to fill the emptiness with alcohol, we begin to discover there is something else available to fill it. For recovering women, *spiritus contra spiritum* can mean the spirit born out of spirits. This is where our spirituality comes from. As Marta says, "I would not have a spiritual life without having traveled the path of addiction."

Spirituality is about staying connected to our source. I often use the lotus flower as a symbol for women's recovery. In a little book called *Inner Beauty: A Book of Virtues,* the lotus is described this way:

> *The main thing about a lotus flower is that it has its root in the mud. It cannot grow without the mud, and yet its petals are pristine. . . . The lotus flower doesn't turn mud into anything. Mud is mud. Yet mud also has nutrients needed to aid the flower's growth. It is the same for us. We are in a situation that we don't like—"in the mud." And yet it is probably the most secure position there is if we could only recognize it, not distort it, and let it "grow us."*[2]

As recovering women, we are like the lotus flower, sending our root down into the mud, our addiction, but always seeking the light. We, like the lotus, don't detach from the mud. Our spirituality is not found by separating ourselves from anything but by staying connected—to the mud, to the truth about our addiction, or to the reality of our life as the source that "grows us."

We begin to make a connection with this spiritual source when we surrender. This is Step One, admitting our powerlessness.

When we surrender, we connect with the spirituality of the Twelve Steps.

When we begin recovery, many of us may be confused about the difference between spirituality and religion. We may think that to be spiritual we have to embrace a certain belief or attend a particular church.

It may be helpful to remember that religion and spirituality can be two separate things. Religion without true spirituality is about beliefs, structures, and rules; it often involves talking about and adopting someone else's spiritual experience. It may not provide a place for the individual to develop her own spiritual understanding and experience.

For many women, a discussion of spirit or spirituality throws us back into the religion of our childhood, an experience that we may feel very distant from or one that had no impact or a negative impact on our lives.

Norma says that her experience with spirituality before she came into the program was very intellectual and matter-of-fact. "I didn't have any religious training. We were a Jewish family. My parents were both immigrants, both spoke Yiddish, but my father, an old-time socialist, was adamantly opposed to any kind of formal religion. 'Spiritual' meant 'religious' to me, and it was outside my realm of experience."

Constance mistrusted the spirituality of the Twelve Steps because it smacked of a distasteful childhood religious experience. "I grew up in a family where three things were genetic: obesity, alcoholism, and fundamentalism," she says. "So when I thought about spirituality I thought about fundamentalism—real good old-fashioned Midwestern rock-ribbed evangelical Christianity. My mother, to stop drinking, became fundamentalist in her religious beliefs; my grandmother was an untreated adult child whose religious beliefs were far more extreme than those of the church to which she belonged; my great-grandmother read the Bible and cried. I wasn't sure I believed in anything when I began recovery."

For other women, religion has always been an important aspect of their lives and continues to shape their recovery process. Shannon, a devout Catholic, finds that her recovery gives life to her religion. "The Twelve Step program gave me an alternative to my old images of God and Jesus," she remembers. "I could personalize God, and that made God real. Recovery gave me my religion back."

Lavonne says the Twelve Steps showed her how to live out her Christian faith. "I was in the county jail on a narcotics charge when I gave my life to the Lord Jesus Christ. The Twelve Steps are one of the things that God used to help me heal. They were the structure of my recovery and a model for my faith."

The religion of our childhood or adulthood can be any of these things and still find expression in recovery: in Twelve Step meetings our individual experience counts—God as we understand God. True spirituality arises from the individual and collective experience of each and all of us. It is all-encompassing; it goes beyond cultural tradition, creed, and sex. Every religious experience and every life experience brings something of value to our spirituality. Many of us lost our sense of spirituality at some time in our lives, yet no matter what our past or present experience, the Twelve Steps give us a chance to rediscover and redefine spirituality for ourselves.

As women, when we talk about spirituality, we often search for new words and images. In describing women's spirituality, I like to use words or phrases like *oneness, wholeness, connection to the universe, belief in something greater than myself, or trust in a higher or deeper part of myself.* Sometimes words like *sacred*—that which has worth within itself and connects to the whole, that which has inherent value yet is connected to everything else—or *profound*—that which arises from the depth of one's being—are most expressive.

Sandy believes that spirituality comes from within. "Knowledge of God begins with knowledge of self," she says. I think she's right. Our spirituality develops in connection to the self as it heals and develops through the Twelve Steps. Our expanding self also unfolds the mystery of spirituality.

Sandy continues, "I think spirituality starts with knowing who we are. Then we expand it by defining our own spirituality—not as men have defined it. That involves looking at what it means to be myself—what it means to be a woman."

Many women feel it is important to describe spiritual experience and their connection to the divine with female metaphors. For some women, spirituality is born from a profound sense of love for oneself that comes from a connection to the image of the goddess and the earth.

Marta finds the images of earth mother and earth goddess, depicted in fertility statues with their feet against their rounded bellies and their big and powerful breasts, potent images for her spirituality. "If we can't love our bodies and ourselves, it is very hard to touch our spirituality," she says. "When we think of the cycles of the moon, the cycles of our menstruation, the cycles of birth and death, we begin to have a tremendous reverence for what it means to bring life into this world. Celebrating motherhood, birth, and creation puts us in touch with the power of the earth that creates and brings forth life. That is the beginning of women's spirituality."

Some think of this feminine Higher Power as the flow of life energy or the natural process of life, birth, death, and decay. Wendy Miller, in her essay "Reclaiming the Goddess," says, "Some speak of Her as a metaphor, some as a spark of divinity, some as igniting creative impulse."[3]

For others, a spirituality that includes male and female is important. This is the case for Darlene. "My spirituality now is more earth-centered and women-centered, but not to the exclusion of men," she says. "I envision a more inclusive spirituality that is not really male or female. I am not willing to insist that God is really a woman and men have been wrong all this time. My Higher Power embodies qualities of both the male and the female, masculine and feminine. But even though I have incorporated some of the goddess consciousness into my spirituality and work, I am troubled by what I see as a separation. I am not an ancient Greek, I am not a druid, I am not an old Celt, thank God! I am a modern woman who is learning new ways of being in the world. While I do believe we need more feminine, life-affirming images of deity—because the spiritual world is so masculine, distorted, and out of balance— I think the feminine images are images of ourselves: not ancient, not images of witchcraft and power over the world and its elements, but feminine images of noncompetitive cooperation and care for the world."

In the process of defining our own spirituality, we may find that the spiritual language of the Steps reflects traditional Christian religious images and practices. Recovering women often struggle with the masculine language in the program and choose to substitute ideas and language that include feminine power.

Maria says, "For those of us who grew up in the Judeo-Christian heritage, God is masculine. So when we think of a Power greater than ourselves, the white-bearded male figure in the clouds comes immediately to mind. I think it is especially important for women to be able to come to a concept of that power that is divorced from gender. It is important to our spirituality that we somehow feminize that power. I have come to believe in a kind of universal, genderless spirit that has nothing to do with my childhood religion. But when I began the Steps it wasn't this way."

Constance approaches the Steps this way: "I have had to do a lot of reworking of the language, like many people of my generation (I'm now in my early fifties) in recovery. The whole concept of God as male—including my childhood concept of God as a rather elderly and robust-looking man with a long white beard—doesn't fit my experience. True spirituality, the source, the creative force that can't be put into words, is beyond gender. Every person reflects equally the spiritual image."

Translating the language and cultural experience of the Twelve Steps for ourselves is an important aspect of recovery. Even the hierarchical structure in the Steps can be a problem for women. Using terms such as "higher" may rob us of a uniquely feminine perspective. Thinking about something "deeper" may be more helpful.

Marta, who was brought up in a fundamentalist, traditional home says, "My family authority structure was hierarchical. The truth is, if I had obeyed or turned my life over to the authority in my family, I'd be dead! So the idea of turning my life over to a hierarchical structure in the Steps was uncomfortable for me. I prefer to think of something not necessarily above me—sometimes it's inside, sometimes outside."

Ruth relates to her Higher Power this way: "I don't think of God as a hierarchical figure, nor as an abstract, higher-up God that I must find on my own," she says. "The 'higher' to me means broader, larger, deeper—not simply me alone using only my energy. I must have other people. The power or energy or whatever you want to call it flows horizontally, from person to person, not from on high."

Women's spirituality often involves ways of being in the world and with each other that are nonhierarchical. Our spirituality expresses interconnection and relationship. Dr. Jan Surrey proposes that our earliest experience of ourselves is relational, that we develop and organize our fundamental concept of self in important relationships. We also deepen and enrich other aspects of this self—our creativity, independence, and assertion—in relationship.[4]

This definition of spirituality from *The Feminine Face of God* is one of my favorites:

> *To a woman, spirituality, or a life of the spirit, implies relationship in its very essence. . . . Relationship that does not separate and divide but connects and brings together spirit and flesh, human beings and other forms of life, God and matter, is precisely what women described to us as the heart of the spiritual in their life.*[5]

Spirituality, God, or Higher Power may not exist above us, or outside of us, but rather in the "between" or "relatedness" we find in meetings, with our sponsor, or in talking about our experience, strength, and hope with another. Darlene says, "I experienced something different in meetings and in myself. I began to experience what I know now as connection, a spiritual experience."

Grace echoes this perception: "What I learned in the program was that I was connected to other people and there was no escaping that. There was nothing to be afraid of because there was no 'alone.' There was nowhere else to go—I wasn't going to go off the planet—I was not without a connection. Being able to be present with and feel the otherness opened my larger sense of relatedness with a Higher Power. The steps opened me up to that new level of relationship."

These experiences awaken and reinforce our inner sense of spirituality, our sense of interconnectedness and relatedness. Our experience of ourselves as spiritual women grows when we sense that the "something beyond" is already within us. When we are vulnerable enough to talk about ourselves with another, when we share our mutual experience, we connect not only with others but with our spiritual self.

Ruth puts it this way: "The universe is primarily moved along creatively by a spirit of mutuality. There is not a father, a God, who oversees and does things. There is, rather, a spirit or force whose essence is particles and dynamics in relation to other particles and dynamics. Things are always connected and interrelated. This spirit or force is a real, present, ongoing power that moves us in right connections and is itself in the essence of the connections. I think it defies the human imagination to imagine what he, she, it is, but that to me is what life force, Higher Power, sacred spirit, God, Goddess is really all about."

Lois asserts simply, "When I say my life is in God's hands, it means in the hands of caring others who are the expressions of divine power. We are here for each other, and through this comes another power."

This other power is the power we have to empower each other. This is available to us in meetings, in the mutual relationship of the sponsor and sponsee, and in joining each other on the path of self-awareness and awakening spirituality.

As Charlotte Spretnak writes in *Ms.,* women's spirituality brings together common themes and concerns: "recognizing the interrelatedness of all life, honoring the dignity of the female, discovering the power of creating ritual, perceiving work for ecological and social justice as a spiritual responsibility, and cultivating sensitivity to diverse multi-cultural experience."[6] These same themes occur over and over again as women talk about spirituality. Our spirituality is about nature, it's about the earth, it's about connectedness, it's about energy, it's about something within us, not just something without.

We may first feel a sense of spirituality in relationship with another person or with our recovery group. As we continue in recovery, our definition of spirituality expands. We discover we are also called into right relation with all of life.

This right relation involves spiritual practice. Grace knows the importance of this in her life. "Practice is the way one is in relation. This includes right relation with the universe, with events, with the day, with nature; it includes practicing mutuality and presence by allowing and encouraging the other to be the 'calling forth.' Practice is a way of being with the wholeness, with events as well as people, with every manifestation, and the appreciation of that in everything," she says.

As Ruth says, "Whether it's washing dishes, gardening, or meditating, it is about staying in this place. Practice forces us to live more fully in the present moment." Eastern religious traditions emphasize practice as the way to enlightenment and the true self, and western traditions call the committed to "practice the presence of God."

When we talk about working the Steps, we are talking about our spiritual practice. Spiritual practice is the process of turning again and again to a discipline or a task, and doing it even when we appear to be going nowhere. The point is to bring ourselves into harmony with the essence of life in the present moment and to express it in all our affairs.

Practice yields serenity. We become more accepting, and we experience a consistent inner peacefulness. We are available to the experience of finding pleasure in everyday things. We are released from the cycle of constant searching and seeking for the quick fix or the high to fill the emptiness. Fulfillment—the real "high"— comes from staying on the path and being present in the moment. We find pleasure in the simple.

"The dailiness is what I love about spirituality," says Grace. "Spiritual experiences are very small and simple; the large ones, if they come at all, are built of lots of smaller ones."

Silence is another simple but important aspect of our spiritual practice. Silence is essential to keeping a balance between our inner life and our outer life. Our world is so congested, and the external world is always coming inward, defiling our sacred place with sound, words, mechanical noise, visual images. A sponsor told me years ago that if I was feeling alone, I was probably lonely for myself. When I heard that, I decided to spend a weekend alone and see what it was like. I turned off the phone and spent the weekend by myself. It was wonderful. What I did, of course, was to rediscover myself.

When we talk about relatedness and connection, we include cultivating relationship and connection with self. When we spend time alone, enjoying the solitude and the quiet, we put the outer self aside and rediscover the inner self. The wholeness that we talk about in recovery is a result of having the inner and the outer balanced and connected so that they reflect each other. In our practice we must spend time cultivating our relationship with ourselves to restore and maintain this balance.

Being in silence and allowing the inner self to be expressed brings us to a profound experience of our spiritual essence. In silence we gain what we call insight—the ability to see within—and rediscover our connection to self. As Buddhist teacher Vimala Thakar writes, in silence we "live in the clarity of knowing who [we] are."[7]

Step Eleven is the way into the silence where we cultivate the flowering of our spiritual self. This Step, "Sought through prayer and meditation to improve our conscious contact with God, *as we understood [God]*," is about deepening our spirituality and creating and maintaining a balance between the inner and outer life.

"This is one of the most challenging steps for me," Marta says. "Conscious contact requires, first of all, being conscious, and that is the true aim of abstinence and of working the Steps. Then it requires intent: I am intentionally choosing to be consciously in contact with whatever I understand my Higher Power to be."

When we seek this conscious contact, it is helpful to remember that there are many forms of meditation and prayer. Our definitions of prayer, meditation, and conscious contact may vary widely.

For Grace, prayer and meditation are ways of being in conversation. She is open to speak and to listen. "Prayer and meditation are like conversation, and that is how we improve our conscious contact," she says. "Prayer reminds me to reach out, to be in a position of asking for help. Prayer is action in relationship."

Ruth describes conscious contact this way: "I know that there is a being that has a plan or purpose for me, in an ego or personal/individual sense. I believe both prayer and meditation are really about being in touch with the spirit that is moving in the universe. They keep me from pulling against that spirit or allowing myself to be cut off from it."

We may also find many different ways to practice conscious contact. Marta's meditation has its own particular expression. "My form of meditation is best served by walking or using the Stairmaster. I accomplish the process of prayer and meditation by ritualistically or repetitively doing some task. I think we've got to remember and encourage women to go back to repetitive tasks like embroidery and knitting, because that is where our conscious process and contact often takes place. In that connection with our own unconscious in the repetition is where we often find our Higher Power to be. I need to find a process that engages the external and the internal in a way that lets me know I've made conscious contact. How do I know I've achieved it? It has a feeling quality to it: there is a calmness that speaks to this elusive term serenity."

Mary Lynn says, "I started painting. That is how I have deepened my conscious contact. My ability to do that has grown and developed over the years." Darlene says she now simply remains open on a daily basis to the unseen and the unknown in her life.

Jackie finds that seeking through prayer and meditation to improve her conscious contact with God (she says Goddess) has been the bulwark of her recovery program. "Once in a while I'll get caught up in tensions and stress and forget it for half a day or so, but I always come back to knowing which side my bread is buttered on—where my source of strength really lies," she says.

Whatever our definition of meditation, prayer, or conscious contact, and however we practice these in our lives, we are seeking through these practices to find something—the will, the way, the inner knowing. As spiritual women these practices also help us to become more centered, grounded, and balanced in order to do the work that the planet needs.

This is also Twelve Step practice—"practic[ing] these principles in all our affairs." Twelve Step practice is about all of us being healers and bringing balance back, first to ourselves and then to the world. We restore balance first in our own lives, working the Steps, healing our addictions, and restoring to balance the unmanageability of our lives. Then we move outward, "to carry the message to others" and "to practice these principles in all our affairs." That is our healing work, and each of us does it in her own way.

Ruth says, "In sobriety one of the absolute delights of my life is experiencing myself as a creature and not simply as a human being.

I am on the earth along with other kinds of creatures, both animal beings and plants, and that increasingly is making me pay attention to what I eat and wear, what I pray for, and who I am with. This sense of connection is a very important part of my spirituality. Along with it comes the idea that I must be involved in struggles for justice. This is what I really believe the spirit is doing in my life and in the world by healing the connections we have on this planet."

When we enter our first Twelve Step meeting, we think we are there simply to overcome our addiction. The Steps may look like the rules of order for sobriety. The surprise comes when we find that the Twelve Steps are a spiritual path, the root that grows our spirituality out of the mud of addiction.

As Katy says, "We're going deeper than alcohol, drugs, or food to see what we are really recovering toward. I've been on a quest," she continues. "I realized, working the Steps, that there is more going on, more to learn here. My business is to do the footwork, to turn it over, and let this God, this inner sensor, take over. I believe there is an alternate reality. I believe there is more going on than my little brain knows about. There are other ways of knowing and perceiving on all levels. My job is to say clean and present so I can have conscious contact."

What started as a process of recovery from addiction becomes a spiritual awakening. "I believe I have had a spiritual awakening as a result of these Steps," says Mary Lynn. "And spiritual awakening is a continual awakening. It's like I am continually coming back to myself. I feel like I've almost come full circle in a way, and that where I'm starting now is where I left off some time ago. Now spirituality is something inside of me. I feel more appreciative of the connection we all have with everything. For me spirituality is a coming back, a reconnecting."

Ruth agrees. "It amazes me to say it, but now I say it without disbelief: I am a very special person who is connected to everything else. Everything, all the energy I put into living life and experiencing the world and seeing the world and understanding the world and changing the world, I now see as part of my spirituality. Spirituality is not an add-on, it is life—it is the way my life is."

Ruth concludes, "In sobriety I've begun to bring back what I would call my own deepest spirituality. I have a deep sense of sacred reality that grounds my being in the world. In sobriety the Steps have to mean tuning into that. Working the Steps becomes a question not of doing something but of connecting to what is. Spirituality and the power of God are like the lotus flower. It was always there, you just didn't see it from your muddy vantage point."

The flowering of our spirituality and our conscious contact with the power of God are not something we add on, but something we awaken to. This sacred reality keeps us rooted in the mud, like the lotus, and nourishes us so that as we become aware we grow, unfold, and blossom into a flower of great beauty.

The Twelve Steps of Alcoholics Anonymous*

1. We admitted we were powerless over alcohol—that our lives had become unmanageable.

2. Came to believe that a Power greater than ourselves could restore us to sanity.

3. Made a decision to turn our will and our lives over to the care of God *as we understood Him.*

4. Made a searching and fearless moral inventory of ourselves.

5. Admitted to God, to ourselves, and to another human being the exact nature of our wrongs.

6. Were entirely ready to have God remove all these defects of character.

7. Humbly asked Him to remove our shortcomings.

8. Made a list of all persons we had harmed, and became willing to make amends to them all.

9. Made direct amends to such people wherever possible, except when to do so would injure them or others.

10. Continued to take personal inventory and when we were wrong promptly admitted it.

11. Sought through prayer and meditation to improve our conscious contact with God *as we understood Him,* praying only for knowledge of His will for us and the power to carry that out.

12. Having had a spiritual awakening as the result of these steps, we tried to carry this message to alcoholics, and to practice these principles in all our affairs.

---

* The Twelve Steps of AA are taken from *Alcoholics Anonymous,* 3d ed., published by AA World Services, Inc., New York, N.Y., 59-60. Reprinted with permission of AA World Services, Inc. (See editor's note on the copyright page.)

Notes

THE STEP BEFORE THE STEPS

1. *Twelve Steps and Twelve Traditions* (New York: Alcoholics Anonymous World Services, 1981), 21.

STEP ONE

1. *Twelve Steps and Twelve Traditions* (New York: Alcoholics Anonymous World Services, 1981), 21.

STEP TWO

1. *Alcohlics Anonymous* (New York: Alcoholics Anonymous World Service, 1976), 47.
2. *Alcoholics Anonymous,* 46.
3. *Twelve Steps and Twelve Traditions* (New York: Alcoholics Anonymous World Services, 1981), 25.
4. *Twelve Steps and Twelve Traditions,* 27.

STEP THREE

1. *Twelve Steps and Twelve Traditions* (New York: Alcoholics Anonymous World Services, 1981), 41.

2. *Alcoholics Anonymous* (New York: Alcoholics Anonymous World Services, 1976), 63.
3. *Alcoholics Anonymous,* 62.
4. *Twelve Steps and Twelve Traditions,* 37.
5. *Twelve Steps and Twelve Traditions,* 35.

STEP FOUR

1. *Twelve Steps and Twelve Traditions* (New York: Alcoholics Anonymous World Services, 1981), 48-49.
2. *Alcoholics Anonymous* (New York: Alcoholics Anonymous World Services, 1976), 67.

STEP FIVE

1. *Twelve Steps and Twelve Traditions* (New York: Alcoholics Anonymous World Services, 1981), 55.
2. *Alcoholics Anonymous* (New York: Alcoholics Anonymous World Services, 1976), 68-70.
3. *Alcoholics Anonymous,* 83.

STEP SIX

1. *Alcoholics Anonymous* (New York: Alcoholics Anonymous World Services, 1976), 60.
2. *Twelve Steps and Twelve Traditions* (New York: Alcoholics Anonymous World Services, 1981), 69.

STEP SEVEN

1. *Alcoholics Anonymous* (New York: Alcoholics Anonymous World

Services, 1976), 76.

2. *Twelve Steps and Twelve Traditions* (New York: Alcoholics Anonymous World Services, 1981), 41.

3. *Alcoholics Anonymous,* 84.

STEP EIGHT

1. *Twelve Steps and Twelve Traditions* (New York: Alcoholics Anonymous World Services, 1981), 77.

2. *Twelve Steps and Twelve Traditions,* 78.

3. *Alcoholics Anonymous* (New York: Alcoholics Anonymous World Services, 1976), 77.

STEP NINE

1. *Alcoholics Anonymous* (New York: Alcoholics Anonymous World Services, 1976), 164.

2. *Alcoholics Anonymous,* 83.

3. Adrienne Rich, *On Lies, Secrets & Silence: Selected Prose 1966-1978.* (New York: Norton, 1979), 183-84.

STEP TEN

1. *Alcoholics Anonymous* (New York: Alcoholics Anonymous World Services, 1976), 84.

2. *Alcoholics Anonymous,* 66.

3. *Twelve Steps and Twelve Traditions* (New York: Alcoholics Anonymous World Services, 1981), 90.

4. Portia Nelson, "Autobiography in Five Short Chapters." In *There's a Hole in My Sidewalk* (Hillsboro, Ore.: Beyond Words Publishing, 1992). ©1992 Portia Nelson. Reprinted with permission.

STEP ELEVEN

1. *Alcoholics Anonymous* (New York: Alcoholics Anonymous World Services, 1976), 63.
2. *Twelve Steps and Twelve Traditions* (New York: Alcoholics Anonymous World Services, 1981), 99.
3. *Twelve Steps and Twelve Traditions,* 98.

STEP TWELVE

1. *Alcoholics Anonymous* (New York: Alcoholics Anonymous World Services, 1976), 58.
2. *Alcoholics Anonymous,* 164.

RELATIONSHIP

1. Jean Baker Miller, "What Do We Mean by Relationship?" (Work in Progress, no. 22, Stone Center for Developmental Services and Studies, Wellesley College, 1986), 1.
2. Stephanie S. Covington and Janet L. Surrey, "The Relational Model of Women's Psychological Development: Implications for Substance Abuse." In *Gender and Alcohol,* edited by S. Wilsnack and R. Wilsnack. (Piscataway, N.J.: Rutgers University, in press).
3. Stephanie S. Covington and Liana Beckett, *Leaving the Enchanted Forest: The Path from Relationship Addiction to Intimacy* (San Francisco: Harper & Row, 1988), 152.
4. Covington and Surrey.
5. Miller, 3.
6. Covington and Surrey.
7. Janet L. Surrey, "Self-in-Relation: A Theory of Women's Development" (Work in Progress, no. 13, Stone Center for Developmental Services and Studies, Wellesley College, 1985), 7.

SEXUALITY

1. Stephanie S. Covington and Janet Kohen, "Women, Alcohol, and Sexuality." *Advances in Alcohol and Substance Abuse* 4 (fall 1984): 41-56.

2. Judith V. Jordan, "Clarity in Connection: Empathic Knowing, Desire, and Sexuality" (Work in Progress, no. 29, Stone Center for Developmental Services and Studies, Wellesley College, 1987), 11.

3. Stephanie S. Covington, *Awakening Your Sexuality: A Guide for Recovering Women and Their Partners* (San Francisco: HarperSanFrancisco, 1991), 219.

SPIRITUALITY

1. "The Bill W. –Carl Jung Letters," *Grapevine* (January 1963): 26.

2. Anthea Church, *Inner Beauty: A Book of Virtues* (Hong Kong: Brahma Humaris Raja Yoga Centre, 1988), 9.

3. Wendy Miller, "Reclaiming the Goddess," *Common Boundary* (March/April 1990): 36.

4. Janet L. Surrey, "Self-in-Relation: A Theory of Women's Development" (Work in Progress, no. 13, Stone Center for Developmental Services and Studies, Wellesley College, 1985).

5. Sherry Ruth Anderson and Patricia Hopkins, *The Feminine Face of God: the Unfolding of the Sacred in Women* (New York: Bantam, 1992), 17.

6. Charlotte Spretnak, "Essay," *Ms.* (April/May 1993): 60.

7. Vimala Thakar, *The Eloquence of Living: Meeting Life with Freshness, Fearlessness & Compassion* (San Rafael, Calif.: New World Library, 1989).

About the Author

Stephanie S. Covington, Ph.D., L.C.S.W., is a nationally recognized clinician, author, organizational consultant, and lecturer. A pioneer in the field of women's issues and addiction and recovery for many years, she has developed an innovative, gender-responsive approach to address the treatment needs of women and girls that results in effective services in public, private, and institutional settings. Her clients include treatment and correctional settings.

Educated at Columbia University and the Union Institute, Dr. Covington is a board-certified Diplomate of the National Association of Social Workers, the American Board of Sexology, and the American Board of Medical Psychotherapists, and is a member of the American Association of Marriage and Family Therapy.

Dr. Covington is based in La Jolla, California, where she is co-director of the Institute for Relational Development and the Center for Gender and Justice. For a list of Dr. Covington's recent articles and descriptions of her current seminars for professionals, visit www.stephaniecovington.com and www.centerforgenderand justice.org or contact Dr. Covington by mail or e-mail:

Institute for Relational Development
Center for Gender and Justice
7946 Ivanhoe Avenue, Suite 201 B
La Jolla, California 92037
sscird@aol.com
www.stephaniecovington.com
www.centerforgenderandjustice.org